MANAGING
Post-Polio
A Guide to Living Well with Post-Polio Syndrome

MANAGING
Post-Polio
A Guide to Living Well with Post-Polio Syndrome

Editor

LAURO S. HALSTEAD, M.D.

Co-Editor

NAOMI NAIERMAN, M.P.A.

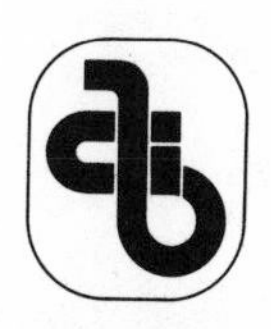

ABI Professional Publications

P.O. Box 5243, Arlington, VA 22205

Paperback edition published by
NRH Press
National Rehabilitation Hospital
Publication Office
102 Irving Street, N.W.
Washington, DC 20010
ISBN 0-9661676-0-0

****

Hardcover edition published by
ABI Professional Publications
P.O. Box 5243
Arlington, VA 22205
ISBN 1-886236-17-8

For my parents

Helen and Gordon Halstead

and my children

Larissa, Christina, and Alexander

Acknowledgments

I am grateful to many people for their help at various stages in the production of this book. Naomi Naierman was helpful throughout the process but particularly in the early stages when this project was getting started. Many people read part or all of the manuscript. Their comments contributed immeasurably to the quality and accuracy of the contents for which I and the other authors are indebted. These people include: James Agre, Augusta Alba, Misty Ash, Ruth Bell, Gabrielle Cjaza, Carrie Clawson, Becky Evans, Hugh Gallagher, Anne Gawne, Selma Harrison-Calmes, Henry Holland, Margo Rowles, Jessica Scheer, Julie Silver, Laura Smith, Daria Trojan, and Tom Walter. Thank you.

I am indebted to Edward A. Eckenhoff for helping establish the NRH Press, which marks its inaugural project with the publication of this book. For technical assistance and support, I want to thank Olga Elizabeth Hayes, Patricia Burton, Robert S. Hartmann, Vassanthi Kolluri, and the publisher, Arthur Brown, who is everyone's fantasy of an ideal publisher. John Rockwood deserves special praise for his generous help and many skills throughout this entire process. Finally, I am grateful to my wife, Jessica Scheer Halstead, for her love and support throughout the many months of gestation and eventual birth of this book.

Managing Post-Polio *was made possible thanks in large part to the generosity of the following organizations:*

THE JM FOUNDATION
ROGER S. FIRESTONE FOUNDATION
THE KIPLINGER FOUNDATION

Contributors

Ruth Wilder Bell, R.N., D.N.Sc.
Past President, the Polio Support Group of Central Maryland
Columbia, MD

Nancy E. Bogg, M.Ed., C.R.C., C.D.M.S., C.C.M.
Rehabilitation Counselor
Cape Elizabeth, ME

Nancy Baldwin Carter, B.A., M.Ed., Psych.
Founder and former Director, Nebraska Polio Survivors Association
Omaha, NE

Hugh Gregory Gallagher, B.A., M.A. Oxon (Honors)
Writer, Historian
Cabin John, MD

Anne C. Gawne, M.D.
Assistant Professor
University of Alabama School of Medicine
Birmingham, AL
Director, Post-Polio Clinic
Roosevelt Warm Springs Institute for Rehabilitation
Warm Springs, GA

Carol J. Gill, Ph.D.
Assistant Professor and Center Director
Chicago Center for Disability Research
Institute on Disability and Human Development
University of Illinois at Chicago
Chicago, IL

Lauro S. Halstead, M.D.
Director, Post-Polio Program
National Rehabilitation Hospital
Clinical Professor of Medicine
Georgetown University School of Medicine
Washington, DC

Stanley L. Lipshultz, J.D., C.P.C.U.
Partner, Lipshultz and Hone, Chtd.
Past President, Polio Society
Past President, Achilles Track Club
Chevy Chase, MD

Kathryn R.B. McGowan, M.A.
Graduate Student in Medical Anthropology
Case Western Reserve University
Cleveland, Ohio

Naomi Naierman, M.P.A.
President, Health Care Ventures
Chevy Chase, MD

Beverly Neway, M.S., C.R.C.
Director, Vocational Rehabilitation Services
National Rehabilitation Hospital
Washington, D.C.

Rhoda Olkin, Ph.D.
Professor of Clinical Psychology
California School of Professional Psychology
Alameda, CA

Liina Paasuke, M.A., C.R.C.
Rehabilitation Counselor
Michigan Jobs Commission Rehabilitation Services
Michigan Polio Network
Co-Facilitator, Post-Polio Connection Support Group
Ann Arbor, MI

Sunny Roller, M.A.
Project Manager, Research Fellow
University of Michigan Medical Center
Ann Arbor, MI

Julie K. Silver, M.D.
Medical Director
Spaulding Neighborhood Rehabilitation Center at Framingham
Instructor in Physical Medicine and Rehabilitation, Harvard Medical School
Consultant in Neurology, Massachusetts General Hospital
Boston, MA

Laura K. Smith, Ph.D., P.T.
Consultant, Post-Polio Clinic
The Institute for Rehabilitation and Research
Houston, TX

Doris Staats, B.A.
Former Member, Board of Directors, The Polio Society
Bethesda, MD

Joyce Ann Tepley, L.M.S.W./A.C.P., L.P.C.
Licensed Clinical Social Worker
Dallas, TX

Tom Walter, B.A.
Volunteer Community Facilitator For Post-Polio Activities for America On-Line (AOL)
Santa Ana, CA

Grace R. Young, M.A., O.T.R.
San Joaquin Valley Rehabilitation Hospital
Fresno, CA

Contents

Introduction

According to the World Health Organization, polio is finally on the verge of extinction. After a run of many millennia, it is now predicted that acute paralytic poliomyelitis will be eliminated from the world not only in our lifetime but, most likely, in the next few years. In this country, the history of polio is much shorter. In fact, the main events were packed into a span of only 39 years—barely two generations—beginning with the first major epidemic in 1916 which was centered in New York City and ending with the announcement on April 12, 1955 that the Salk vaccine was safe and effective. Since then, for most Americans, the epidemics have sunk into oblivion and polio no longer refers to a disease but a vaccine. Yet, for many thousands of us, the legacy of our nation's brief rendezvous with polio is still very much a part of our personal histories and daily lives.

Beginning with our first encounter with this summer plague, many polio survivors tell a story of struggle and triumph: the sudden, random onset of paralysis, the gradual restoration of strength, seemingly as a result of individual willpower, and finally, achieving a full and productive life, which led us to believe we had put polio behind us. This story, for most, was made possible by denying our disability and the reality of what was lost and the life that might have been. While this kind of denial is not unique to polio, its unyielding persistence is unusual. Virtually every polio survivor I have met has displayed an element of this self-deception. Until recently, most of us tended to avoid other polio survivors and even persons with disabilities. We knew we weren't physically normal, but, if we thought about it at all, we considered ourselves as inconvenienced, not disabled. By retraining the muscles that remained, we felt we could do just about anything, even become President of the United States, like Franklin Delano Roosevelt.

It has now been almost two decades since the term post-polio syndrome (PPS) entered our lives. Even though the occurrence of new weakness and other symptoms several decades after acute polio was described many years ago in the medical literature, our experience with these symptoms was new and unexpected. For many of us, the denial was still intact, which made understanding and accepting the new changes all the more difficult. As we began to acknowledge the fact that we *were disabled*, we were overcome by feelings of anger, bitterness, and despair.

Fortunately, the feelings did not stop there. The knowledge and skills of how to not just endure but prevail, to paraphrase Faulkner, were still intact. Our shared history of knowing how to overcome adversity led us to take action that, once again, turned our lives around and made us feel proud to be called *survivors*. One step was to stimulate the medical community to take our new health problems seriously. Over the years, this has led to a significant increase in the attention given to polio by researchers and clinicians leading to a more precise definition of PPS, a better understanding of the possible causes, and the development of more rational and effective strategies for its management.

Another step was reaching out to others, specifically others who had polio and were experiencing similar new problems; but it wasn't just to find others that hundreds of support groups emerged from nowhere overnight. It was, more importantly, part of a journey of self-discovery. In my own case, it was only after I joined a local support group and began talking with other polio survivors that I started to grieve the body I had lost more than three decades earlier. Although I still have not made peace with my disability, and probably never will, I am getting better at incorporating it into my life and the person I am. One of the reasons it is hard to find this peace is that my disability keeps changing: as I age, as I develop other infirmities, as it progresses.

This leads to one of the goals for this book. It was written and edited partly to *help me* deal better with my own unique disability and, at the same time, to help the many thousands of other polio survivors in this country and around the world deal more effectively with their unique version of polio disability. Despite a lot of hard work, this book is not the last word on PPS. That book will have to wait. It may be many more years—maybe never. In my own mind, I am still not entirely certain what PPS is. There is no question, however, *there are new symptoms*, most importantly, new weakness, related to the earlier paralysis—whether that paralysis was catastrophic or passed like a shadow in the night. What I am not clear about is whether there is a single entity that we wisely label PPS or several entities that, out of ignorance and for convenience, we call PPS until our knowledge becomes more sophisticated. In the meantime, there is no doubt that giving the symptoms a name has been helpful. Without a name, it does not exist for practical purposes: people cannot talk about it, scientists cannot study it, and authors cannot write articles and books to educate and inform others.

Another goal in writing this book was to distill and summarize *in lay terms* the wealth of information presented at conferences and published in the medical and allied health literature over the past 10 to 15 years. In the process of describing clearly and accurately what is felt to be most important, it is sometimes necessary to opt for fewer details and technical explanations. For readers who would like more information on a specific topic, there are references and resources listed by chapter in the Appendix. While a reader–friendly book is a worthy goal, not many friends or other readers are likely to purchase it if the cost is too high. With this in mind, we were fortunate to obtain outside funding from three foundations (The JM Foundation, Roger S. Firestone Foundation, and Kiplinger Foundation) to keep the final price of the book reasonable, and hopefully, within reach of all who would like to obtain a copy.

A third goal was to give these pages a tone of authenticity. Almost all of the authors are polio survivors or persons who have had extensive experience working or living with polio survivors. In addition, the Appendix contains first person accounts by seven individuals in various stages of their lifetime struggles and triumphs with polio and post-polio syndrome. These stories provide eloquent testimony to the many ways people have prevailed in the face of ongoing disability. These experiences complement in more personal and human terms the material presented in the earlier chapters of the book. Finally, a goal of all of us who contributed to this volume was to provide practical information and useful strategies for managing PPS with the hope of helping each reader achieve a healthier and more enjoyable life.

Lauro S. Halstead, M.D.
February, 1998

1

Acute Polio and Post-Polio Syndrome

LAURO S. HALSTEAD

Most of us think of polio as an epidemic disease. Yet, it wasn't until the end of the 19th century when the first epidemic was recorded in Stockholm, Sweden. Before that, polio made many isolated appearances throughout history, beginning in the time of the ancient dynasties of Egypt. One example, and maybe the earliest case of recorded poliomyelitis, was discovered by archaeologists in an Egyptian mummy who died sometime around 3700 BC. Another example dating from 1400 BC shows a young Egyptian priest in a stone carving leaning on a staff with a shortened, deformed foot in the characteristic pose of a polio-affected limb.

The first comprehensive descriptions of polio in the medical literature were published in the 1800s by two European physicians, Drs. Jacob von Heine and Karl Medin from Germany and Sweden, respectively. For a time, polio was known as Heine-Medin disease. In America, there were sporadic reports of poliomyelitis as early as 1841, but the first U.S. epidemic did not occur until 1894 near Rutland, Vermont. By 1913, polio had appeared in every state and province of the United States and Canada, afflicting over 25,000 children and adults.

It was not until 1916, however, that polio took center stage even briefly in our national awareness. In that year, the first major U.S. epidemic occurred. More than 9,000 cases were reported in New York City alone, resulting in 2,400 deaths and panic in the streets. The vast majority of those affected were under the age of five years, which led to the name "infantile paralysis." Although scientists had identified the poliovirus in 1908, there was wild speculation by the lay public about the cause of this frightening disease, including everything from "stray cats to doctors' beards to radio waves."

Five years after the epidemic of 1916, Franklin Delano Roosevelt contracted "infantile paralysis" at the age of 39 years and the course of polio history was changed forever. Although his legs were badly paralyzed, FDR never lost faith that he might walk again. With remarkable courage and a flair for denial, Roosevelt continued his political career and private life masking his disability. Over the years and during his frequent visits to Warm Springs (the great polio Mecca he established in southern Georgia), FDR stayed in touch with other polio survivors and actively supported the search for better treatments and a vaccine. This commitment ultimately led to the creation in 1937 of the National Foundation for Infantile Paralysis (later known as the March of Dimes). During the next two decades, the March of Dimes played a central role in raising the money necessary to develop the polio vaccines.

During the 1930s, 1940s, and 1950s, the polio epidemics seemed unstoppable. As they grew in size, they became more deadly, creating a climate of fear and awe that is difficult to imagine today. From 1951 to 1955, approximately 40,000 cases were reported each year, with infections striking increasingly at older children and young adults. Starting in 1951, an effort was made to improve the accuracy of diagnosis and to report cases as either paralytic or nonparalytic. Perhaps partly because of this effort, the next year, 1952, became the largest epidemic year on record when almost 60,000 cases were reported. Of these, more than one-third had paralysis and more than 3,000 persons died.

By 1953, more American children died of paralytic poliomyelitis than any other communicable disease. Unlike the current AIDS epidemic, polio haunted everyone: families stayed at home, swimming pools were closed, public events were canceled. Children, in particular, were at risk, especially during the hot summer months. As one observer commented, polio seemed to seek out children, the most vulnerable among us.

At all ages, polio affected males slightly more than females. In the middle and upper classes, paralytic polio was more common than in the lower classes. The explanation for this socioeconomic difference was that children in lower classes, which tend to have more crowding and poorer sanitation, were more likely to be exposed to the virus at a young age when the illness was generally milder and lifetime immunity (natural protection) was acquired.

All races contracted the disease in proportion to their representation in each socioeconomic class, although in the late epidemics the death rate was higher among African Americans, who often had less access to specialized treatments, such as the iron lung. In early epidemics, when no treatment existed, death rates among the races were similar.

Epidemic poliomyelitis was found throughout the United States in rural and urban settings alike, with particularly high rates in the growing suburbs of post-World War II America. Epidemics peaked and ebbed from year to year and were usually explained in two ways: (1) by environmental conditions that either encouraged or discouraged transmission of the disease and (2) by variations in the strength of different strains of the poliovirus passing through a population. Even though an enormous amount of scientific information is known about polio, it remains a curious fact that there is still no fully satisfactory explanation of why and where epidemics occurred in any given year.

THE POLIO VACCINES

On April 12, 1955—10 years to the day after FDR's death—it was announced in a dramatic national radio and television broadcast that the Salk vaccine was both safe and effective. It was a triumphant moment for U.S. medicine and brought enormous pride and relief to the American people. To use a metaphor of the time, the war against polio was over. Newspapers carried full-page headlines, "Polio Conquered," and "Victory Over Polio." American technology had won. Towns across the country held parades with marching bands and signs reading, "No More Polio," "Thank you, Dr. Salk," and "Our children are safe again."

Salk immunization, given by injection, uses killed or inactivated virus particles. The vaccine is usually called IPV for inactivated polio vaccine. Because the virus is killed, the vaccine is extremely safe and cannot cause new cases of polio. Six years after Jonas Salk's extraordinary triumph, Albert Sabin's vaccine became available in 1961 following testing in Russia. The Sabin vaccine uses live, but attenuated or "weakened" virus particles, and is given by mouth. For this reason, it is often called OPV or oral polio vaccine. Because the weakened OPV virus can be "passed" from person to person, thus immunizing many other individuals with a single dose, the Sabin vaccine is considered superior to the Salk. However, it does have the great disadvantage of producing paralytic polio in an extremely small number of recipients (approximately 1 out of 700,000 individuals after the first immunization).

Following the widespread use of the vaccines, the incidence of polio dropped dramatically in the mid and late 1950s. During the next two decades, polio almost disappeared. In 1979, 24 years after the introduction of the Salk vaccine, the last case of paralytic polio caused by a live wild virus was reported in the United States.

Tragically, despite this extraordinary accomplishment, acute polio was still being reported until the mid-1990s. Approximately 10 to 12 new cases of paralytic polio were caused each year by the weakened virus in the Sabin vaccine. Most of the affected individuals became paralyzed because of an immune deficiency (an abnormality of the body's defense mechanism). Such deficiencies reduce the body's ability to fight infections, making it easier, even for weakened viruses, to gain a foothold and cause serious illness.

Because vaccine-related polio is completely preventable with the use of the Salk vaccine, the U.S. government changed its policy in 1996. It now recommends that two immunizations with IPV be given initially, followed at later intervals by two doses of OPV. In theory, this combination provides the advantages of both vaccines.

Meanwhile, on the global level, the efforts of the World Health Organization, Rotary International, and other organizations to eradicate polio from the world by the year 2000 are beginning to pay off. During 1996, the number of officially reported polio cases was under 4,000. Using "national immunization days," which are the main tool of the polio eradication campaign, many countries have been able to completely eliminate polio. On a single day, in January 1997, approximately 127 million children in India were vaccinated against polio in what is believed to be the largest health event ever organized by a country. If polio is eradicated from the world, it will join smallpox as only the second disease humankind has successfully eliminated from the globe.

THE FOUR STAGES OF POLIO

Historically, polio has been divided into three fairly distinct stages: acute illness, period of recovery, and stable disability. In the early 1980s, clinicians and researchers began to realize that there was a fourth stage characterized by the onset of new symptoms related to the original polio attack. This stage has been described by various terms, including "the late effects of polio," "post-polio sequelae," "post-polio progressive muscular atrophy," "post-polio muscle dysfunction," and "post-polio syndrome." The names "post-polio muscle dysfunction" and "post-polio progressive muscular atrophy" emphasize abnormal muscle function. This narrow focus makes these terms more appropriate for research. By contrast, "post-polio syndrome" or PPS is more broadly defined, making it more practical for clinical purposes. In addition, PPS has been widely used in the medical and lay literature for many years. For these reasons, PPS is used in this book.

Figure 1.1 shows the typical course for the three traditional stages of paralytic polio as well as the beginning of Stage IV or PPS. These health and functional changes are based on the acute and chronic polio experience of a group of persons evaluated at the post-polio clinic in Houston, Texas.

Stage I: Acute Illness

The onset of polio is characterized by a mild fever, headache, sore throat, diarrhea or vomiting, and malaise (a general sense of not feeling well). Initial symptoms are similar to many other viral illnesses. In the great majority of individuals, these symptoms are gone within two or three days. In a small minority, less than 5 percent, the symptoms are more severe, reflecting a viral invasion of the central nervous system (CNS), which consists of the spinal cord and brain. Infection of the CNS results in a sharp escalation of symptoms with high fever, stiff neck, severe headache, and muscle pains. In some, the disease stops there and no weakness or paralysis ever occurs. In others, approximately 1 percent to 2 percent of the affected, the infection continues to spread, producing variable amounts of muscle paralysis or weakness in the limbs, trunk, and

Figure 1.1 Natural History of Polio

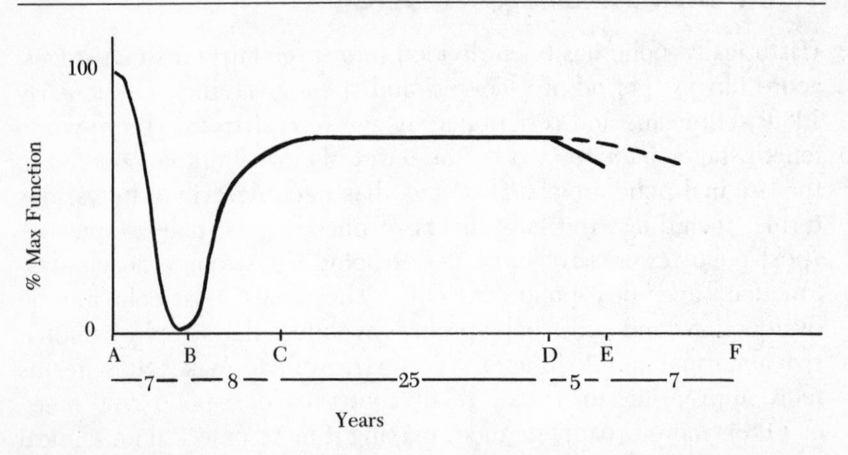

Legend: Health and functional changes showing the four stages of polio for 132 individuals with PPS evaluated at the post-polio clinic in Houston, Texas. A = birth; B = onset of acute polio or Stage I (average age of seven years); B to C = period of recovery or Stage II (an average of eight years); C to D = maximum recovery and period of neurologic and functional stability or Stage III (an average of 25 years); D = onset of PPS or Stage IV (B to D an average of 33 years); E = time of clinic evaluation (D to E an average of five years); F = death (E to F: unknown). Dashed line = projected course without PPS.

even the face and neck. During the large epidemics of the 1940s and 1950s, roughly 12 percent of those who developed acute paralytic poliomyelitis died from breathing or swallowing complications.

Stage II: Period of Recovery or Convalescence

Recovery begins as soon as an individual's temperature returns to normal and the other symptoms subside. This stage can last from weeks to years, depending on the severity of involvement and age at onset. Persons who contract polio as children or infants and have extensive paralysis take the longest time to recover. During this period, individuals usually begin an intensive program of rehabilitation in hospital or home with the goal of strengthening and retraining weakened muscles and learning to regain lost function. For the group of persons shown in Figure 1.1, the average length of Stage II was eight years.

Stage III: Stable Disability or the Stage of Chronicity

Stage III begins when a person reaches a plateau of maximum recovery of strength and stamina. The precise time when this stage starts may be hard to determine, especially if the individual is still growing and changing developmentally or is undergoing reconstructive surgery to enhance strength and function. Despite these difficulties, most people have a general idea when their recovery was complete.

Stage IV: Post-Polio Syndrome

The third stage of polio lasts indefinitely for many individuals, perhaps for the majority who had paralytic polio. For 20 percent to 40 percent of individuals, the stage of stable disability ends and Stage IV or PPS begins with the onset of new weakness, which is often accompanied by other symptoms, such as fatigue, pain in muscles or joints, and decreased function. For the individuals in Figure 1.1, Stage III lasted an average of 25 years. Stage IV began, on average, 33 years after the acute onset of polio. A similar interval is found in other studies, but the range has been reported to extend from two decades to eight decades.

DEFINITION OF POST-POLIO SYNDROME

Post-polio syndrome is a *neurologic disorder* that produces a cluster of symptoms in individuals who had paralytic polio many years earlier. Because these symptoms tend to occur together, they are called a syndrome. Typically, these problems occur after a period of functional and neurological stability of *at least 15 years* following the initial episode of polio and include new weakness, fatigue, decreased endurance and loss of function. Some researchers also add pain as part of the syndrome, especially in muscles and joints. Less commonly, the symptoms include muscle atrophy (shrinkage), breathing and swallowing difficulties, and cold intolerance. Some of the symptoms (e.g., weakness, fatigue, and atrophy) appear to be caused by a progressive degeneration or impairment of motor units (Figure 1.2). Other symptoms (e.g., muscle and joint pain) are more likely the result of excessive wear and tear on different parts of the musculoskeletal system, although this wear and tear can be brought on or made worse when muscles become weaker.

Figure 1.2 The Motor Unit

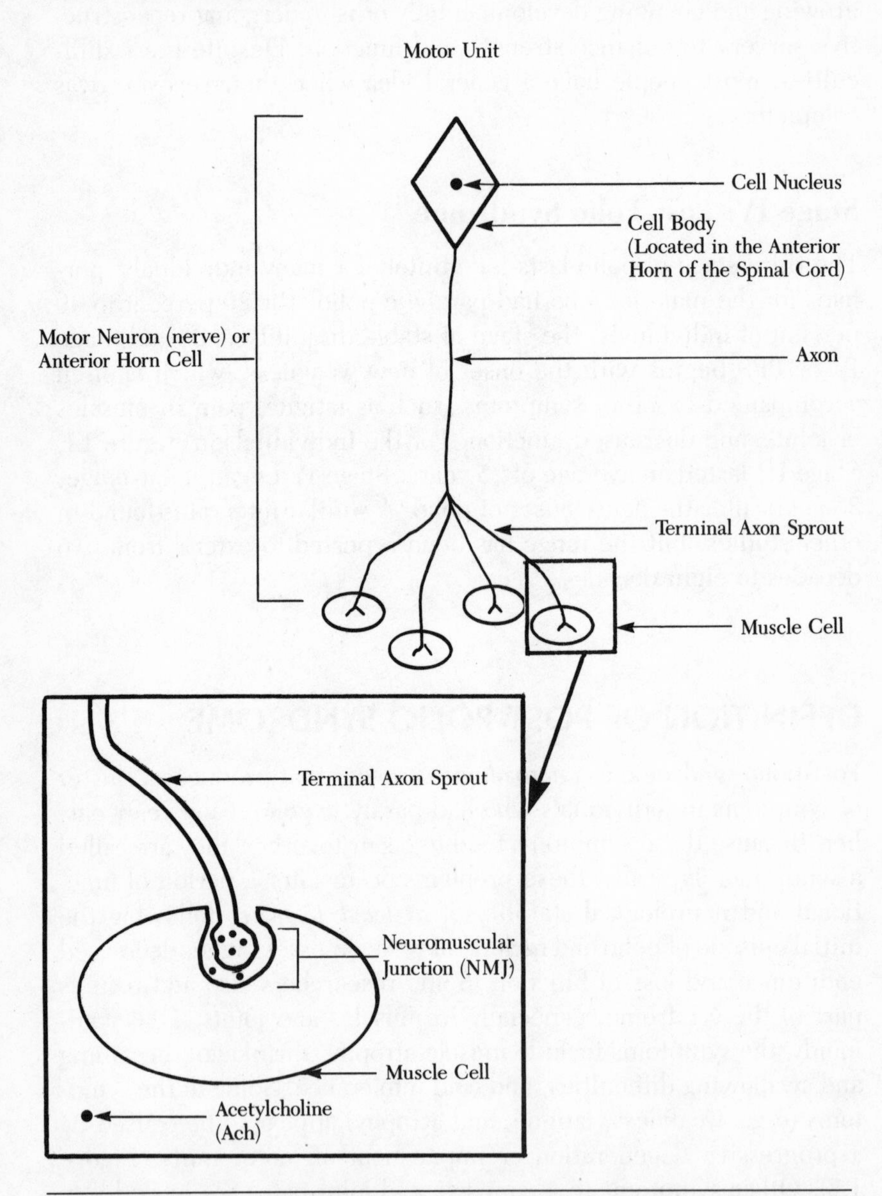

Legend: The motor unit consists of a motor nerve or anterior horn cell (cell body, axon and axon sprouts) and all the muscle cells stimulated by that nerve. The cell body (which regulates the motor nerve functions) is located in the anterior horn of the spinal cord. Axons are just short or long enough to reach the muscles they stimulate to contract. Axons that supply muscles in the legs can be three or more feet in length. The insert shows a close-up view of the neuromuscular junction. This is where the terminal axon sprout stimulates the muscle cell to contract by releasing the chemical acetylcholine (Ach).

The percentage of new health and functional problems reported by persons evaluated in several post-polio clinics is listed in Table 1.1. The most common problems are fatigue, weakness, and pain in muscles and joints. The new weakness is located in muscles previously affected by polio as well as in muscles thought to be *unaffected* by the original illness. At first glance, the phenomenon of "unaffected" muscles becoming weak seems contradictory but, in fact, is well known. Usually, it means that the polio was so mild in those muscles at the time of the original illness that the individual, as well as health care professionals, were unaware of any polio involvement in those particular limbs. Yet, there was enough loss of motor neurons that after many years of overuse new weakness developed. The most common new functional problems include increased difficulty in walking, climbing stairs, and dressing—activities that require repetitive muscular contractions.

THE HISTORY OF POST-POLIO SYNDROME

For more than 100 years, the late effects of polio have been known to occur in some individuals many years after their initial illness. The first descriptions appeared in 1875 in the French medical literature. The cases involved three young men who had paralytic polio

Table 1.1 New Health and Functional Problems

Symptom	Percent (Range)
HEALTH PROBLEMS	
Fatigue	86–87
Muscle pain	71–86
Joint pain	71–79
Weakness	
Previously affected muscles	69–87
Previously unaffected muscles	50–77
Cold intolerance	29–56
Atrophy	28–39
ADL PROBLEMS[1]	
Walking	64–85
Stair climbing	61–83
Dressing	16–62

[1]ADL = Activities of daily living

in infancy and developed significant new weakness and atrophy as young adults. These new problems occurred in muscles previously affected by polio and in muscles thought to be spared. All of the subjects had physically demanding jobs that required strength and repetitive activities. In a commentary on one of the cases, the great 19th-century French neuropathologist, Jean Martin Charcot, suggested several hypotheses for these changes. He believed an initial disease of the spinal cord (such as polio) might leave some individuals more susceptible to a subsequent spinal disorder. He also hypothesized that the new weakness was caused by overuse of the involved muscles. His observations are surprisingly relevant to the current understanding of PPS.

After those initial reports, there was only sporadic interest in the late effects of polio for many decades. In the century following Charcot's observations, fewer than 35 published reports appeared, describing less than 250 cases. As with the first subjects, these reports described new problems that included weakness, atrophy, and fasciculations (involuntary muscle contractions or twitching), occurring up to 71 years after an attack of paralytic polio.

Why these after effects of polio remained an obscure and largely unexplored area of medicine until recently is not clear. Few diseases are as widely prevalent in the world or have been as intensively investigated as polio. Because of the rapid and dramatic onset of symptoms, polio was viewed as a classic example of an acute viral infectious disease. As a result, most of the scientific energy and resources were directed at early management and prevention with virtually no research into long-term sequelae or after effects. Until recently, medical textbooks classified paralytic polio as a *static* or stable neurological disease.

With widespread use of the vaccines, polio quickly became a medical oddity in the industrialized world; interest and funding in polio-related problems waned. However, polio and its complications only *appeared* to have been defeated. Because the major epidemics occurred in the 1940s and 1950s and new neurologic changes appeared 30 years to 40 years later, many thousands of polio survivors did not begin to experience new problems related to their polio until the late 1970s and early 1980s.

By sheer weight of numbers, persons experiencing PPS finally started attracting widespread attention in the early 1980s. The term "post-polio syndrome" was coined at about the time of the first International Post-Polio Conference at Warm Springs, Georgia, in May 1984. In the intervening years, there has been a marked increase in the attention focused on PPS by researchers and clinicians, leading to a more precise definition, a better understanding of possible causes, and development of more effective management.

EPIDEMIOLOGICAL ASPECTS OF POST-POLIO SYNDROME

Accurate numbers of Americans who had paralytic poliomyelitis are not available and probably never will be. There is no national registry of persons who had polio. Also, there is no way, after all these years, to compile accurate figures from state and local health departments. The best estimate is based on data from the government's National Center for Health Statistics, which conducts a National Health Interview Survey each year. This survey collects data from a random sample of the U.S. population regarding various health and disability issues. In 1987, surveyors specifically asked questions about the number of persons who were given a diagnosis of poliomyelitis with or without paralysis. Based on the results of this survey, the Center calculated slightly more than 1.63 million polio survivors. Of these, 641,000 (39.2 percent) persons had paralytic polio; 833,000 (51 percent) had non-paralytic polio; and 160,000 (9.8 percent) didn't know. Unfortunately, some of these data have been miscopied or misrepresented and then erroneously published in the medical literature as fact. The most common error is the statement citing 1.63 million persons with paralytic polio when the correct estimate is really 641,000 as cited above.

The latter figure, however, is based on a survey conducted 10 years ago. Since then, it has been estimated that 5 percent to 10 percent of the polio population has died, which means the current number of survivors is closer to 600,000. How many of these 600,000 persons with paralytic polio have PPS is unknown. Several studies indicate a large number, perhaps 60 percent or more, is experiencing one or more new difficulties related to old polio, such as muscle aches and joint pains. However, *the number with PPS* (new weakness with or without other symptoms many years after acute polio) is undoubtedly smaller, probably in the range of 20 percent to 40 percent. Using these figures, it is estimated that approximately 120,000 persons to 240,000 persons in this country are currently experiencing symptoms of PPS.

THE RELATION OF ACUTE POLIO TO POST-POLIO SYNDROME

The word *poliomyelitis* comes from the Greek, *polios*, gray, and *myelos*, marrow, and the English ending, *itis*, inflammation. When seen in cross-section, the spinal cord has both white and gray areas. The poliovirus produces an inflammation of the gray marrow portion of the spinal cord located in the front or anterior part of the cord (Figure 1.3). This area is called the *anterior horn*; the nerve cells clustered there are called *anterior horn cells*. As poliovirus attacks almost exclusively the motor nerve cells in the anterior horn of the spinal cord, physicians sometimes refer to polio as an anterior horn cell disease or AHCD.The acute infection is caused by one of three types or strains of polioviruses called Types I, II and III. Type I is often responsible for the most severe paralysis. These types are sometimes confusing as the same word is used to describe the clinical types of polio, e.g., spinal, bulbar, or spinal-bulbar. However, the *virus type* is *not* related in any way to the *clinical type* of illness. After an individual has been infected with one strain of virus, the body develops lifelong immunity protecting it from reinfection with that type of virus ever again. As the three types of viruses are immunologically distinct (because of differences in their protein coats), infection with one does not provide protection from the others. This phenomenon explains why some individuals have had polio twice and why, in theory, it is even possible to have it three times.

Acute infection occurs when the virus enters the body through the mouth from water or food contaminated with feces. Following multiplication in the tissues of the throat and intestine, the virus passes harmlessly from the gut or penetrates the intestinal wall and travels in the blood to all parts of the body. The great majority of infected individuals have no symptoms or experience a self-limited illness characterized by fever and gastrointestinal upset for several days. In one percent to two percent of the population, the virus

Figure 1.3 Cross-section of the Spinal Cord

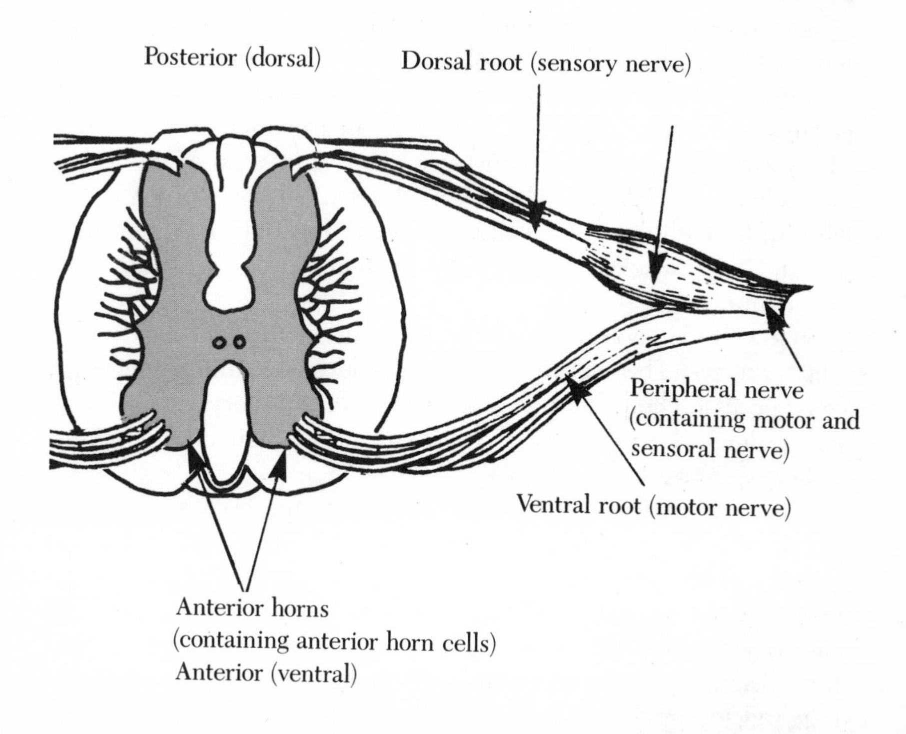

Legend: The cross-section of the spinal cord showing both white and gray areas. The anterior horn appears gray due to the clustering of anterior horn cells. The white matter consists of nerves covered with a whitish insulation material called myelin. The peripheral nerve shown here is a "mixed" nerve and is formed by a posterior (sensory) nerve and an anterior (motor) nerve. Some peripheral nerves have only a sensory component and others only a motor component.

invades the spinal cord by traveling up the motor neurons to the anterior horns, where it can result in a variable amount of paralysis.

Regardless of the extent of paralysis, however, the virus is widely distributed, typically infecting over 95 percent of the motor neurons in the spinal cord and many other cells in the brain as well. Following this invasion, cells die or shed the virus and regain a normal or near-normal appearance. Whether these recovered motor neurons are more likely to sustain injury or begin to malfunction later in life is unknown. If they are more easily injured or overworked, it might provide one explanation for the new weakness in those with PPS.

To gain a better understanding of what happens to nerves and muscles after a bout of acute polio, it is useful to review some basic anatomy. Figure 1.2 shows a motor nerve cell or motor neuron (comprising a cell body, a long tentacle called an axon, and axon sprouts). The sprouts or rootlets, which branch out at the end of the axons, are called terminal axon sprouts. Each terminal axon sprout stimulates an individual muscle cell to contract. Together the motor neuron and the muscle cells supplied by that neuron are called the motor unit.

Following an acute attack of polio, some motor neurons die and others survive. The ones that survive can develop additional terminal axon sprouts. Their function is to reconnect (reinnervate) nerves to muscle fibers left "orphaned" by the death of their original motor neurons (Figure 1.4, B and C).

In a sense, the growth of axon sprouts is the body's effort at a rescue mission to keep as many muscle cells alive and working as possible. This compensatory process allows an uninfected or recovered motor neuron to adopt as many as seven, eight, or even ten additional muscle fibers for every muscle cell stimulated by that nerve originally. This process means a single motor neuron that was designed to supply 1,000 muscle fibers might eventually be redesigned to stimulate as many as *10,000 fibers* or a total of *9,000 extra* muscle cells beyond its original capacity. Thus, the size of many motor units *increases significantly* after acute polio, resulting in what are called *giant motor units*. These giant motor units make it possible for a few motor neurons to do the work of many (Figure 1.4, C).

In addition to the extra sprouting that makes giant motor units, the other major mechanism that produces a return of strength is *muscle cell hypertrophy* (enlargement), which develops in response to exercise. These mechanisms of compensation (hypertrophy and axon sprouting) explain how persons experienced what appeared to be a miracle cure and could go from bed to wheelchair to walking over a period of 6 months to 12 months. During the ensuing interval of stable strength and endurance (Figure 1.1, Stage III), it appears to the individual that recovery has been completed. Yet, as it turns out, the compensatory mechanisms keep right on working. If old

Figure 1.4 Motor Neurons and Muscle Cells Before and After Polio

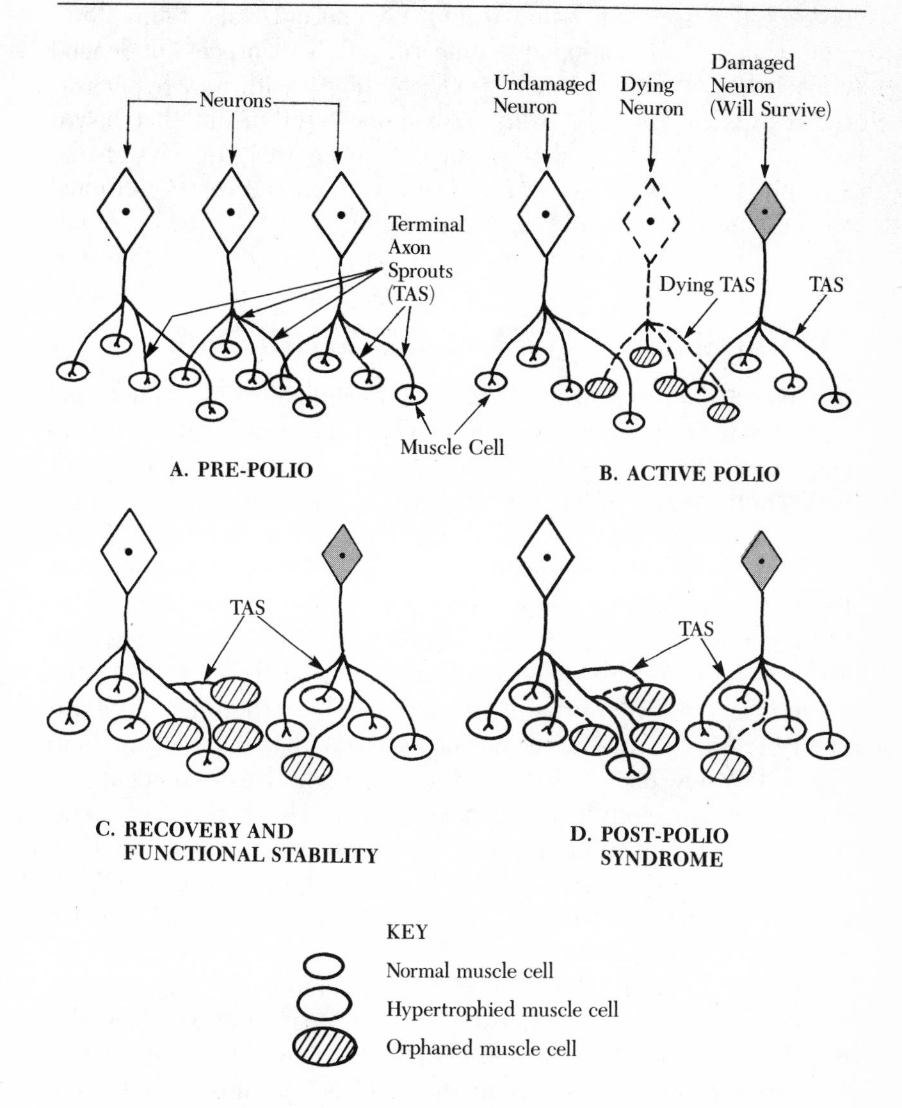

Legend: A = pre-polio; three normal motor neurons and the muscle cells they supply; B = acute stage of polio. The motor neuron on the left is not invaded by the poliovirus and remains undamaged. The middle neuron is infected and dies and the entire nerve disintegrates. The muscle cells (shaded) become "orphaned" or "stranded." The motor neuron on the right is infected with the virus but survives; C = the stages of recovery and functional stability. The orphaned muscle cells are "adopted" or re-connected to the surviving motor neurons by the growth of new terminal axon sprouts (TAS) creating "giant motor units." When these muscles cells become re-connected and start working again, the individual regains lost strength. Note the enlarged or hypertrophied muscle cells which develop in response to exercise. These enlarged cells also help increase an individual's strength; and D = PPS. In the two remaining motor neurons, some terminal axon sprouts are dying and new ones have grown. However, not all orphaned muscle cells become reconnected to motor neurons, leading to new weakness.

terminal axon sprouts drop off (producing a disconnection between nerves and muscles or *denervation*), new sprouts take their place (producing a reconnection or *reinnervation*). This process of denervation balanced with reinnervation, combined with new hypertrophy, results in a *steady state* or dynamic equilibrium that helps maintain a constant level of strength. When this steady state is disrupted after many years, a critical threshold is crossed and new weakness occurs, marking the onset of PPS.

THE CAUSE(S) OF POST-POLIO SYNDROME

No universal agreement exists about the cause of PPS. A growing consensus is developing among researchers, however, that the major symptom of PPS, new progressive weakness, is caused by a degeneration of the motor units. This explanation is not surprising because we know already that the motor unit is the primary target of the poliovirus during the original illness. To take this understanding one step further, data from a large number of studies by many researchers suggest that motor unit degeneration may occur at three separate levels reflecting three different defects or abnormalities. One abnormality is at the level of the motor neuron where there is a deterioration of the terminal axon and old sprouts that drop off are not replaced by new ones. A second abnormality involves a defect at the level of the neuromuscular junction or NMJ. This is the site where each motor neuron stimulates individual muscle cells to contract by releasing a chemical called acetylcholine or Ach (Figure 1.2). The current hypothesis is that too little Ach is made or released, resulting in a defect that causes diminished contraction of the muscle or no contraction at all. (This defect can be temporarily improved in some individuals using pyridostigmine or Mestinon® which works by enhancing the effect of Ach at the neuromuscular junction.) A third abnormality may occur at the level of the muscle cell itself which results in decreased strength when the muscle contracts. How much muscle cell changes contribute to the overall picture of new weakness is uncertain.

Does this complete our understanding about the cause of PPS? Unfortunately not, as the underlying reason why motor units start to fail *in the first place* is still a mystery. Among many theories, probably the most likely is that of *overuse*. This theory is based on the assumption that the greatly enlarged motor units that drive post-polio muscles have labored for decades under an increased burden just to maintain everyday activities. This increased burden or over-use, the theory goes, eventually results in a degeneration of the motor unit after a certain number of years.

In addition to overuse, numerous other hypotheses have been proposed to explain the progressive weakness of PPS. These hypotheses include premature aging of the motor units, persistence of poliovirus fragments, an autoimmune process (where the body attacks itself), environmental toxins that injure motor neurons, changes in the spinal cord (such as scarring), muscle overuse, and hormone deficiencies. While some of these theories seem plausible and none have been completely excluded, not enough evidence exists to justify strong support of any of these other hypotheses at the present time.

Of all the symptoms of PPS, new weakness is the easiest to study and, thus, has stimulated the most research. The results from this research have provided a better understanding of this symptom than any other aspect of PPS. Ironically, the symptom of fatigue is more common than new weakness in most studies but, because it is more difficult to investigate, much less is known about the cause. In addition, fatigue is an imprecise term with several meanings. In the context of PPS, people are sometimes referring to muscle fatigability or the muscle fatigue that occurs with repetitive muscle contractions. This condition is easily demonstrated in a weak muscle when it is given a small amount of resistance and does not produce as much force on the fifth, seventh, or tenth contraction as it does on the first. This phenomenon is called *peripheral* fatigue and is probably caused by motor unit degeneration and the same mechanisms that produce new weakness.

In addition to peripheral fatigue, another type is known as central fatigue. For many individuals, this type is the most disabling symptom of PPS. It is characterized by the rapid onset of mild to extreme tiredness, generalized headache, difficulty in concentrating, and general malaise. The origin of central fatigue is unknown, but one possibility is that it may also be caused by motor unit abnormalities—either at the level of the degenerating terminal axons or perhaps in the muscle itself, or both.

Figure 1.5 Side View of the Brain and Brainstem

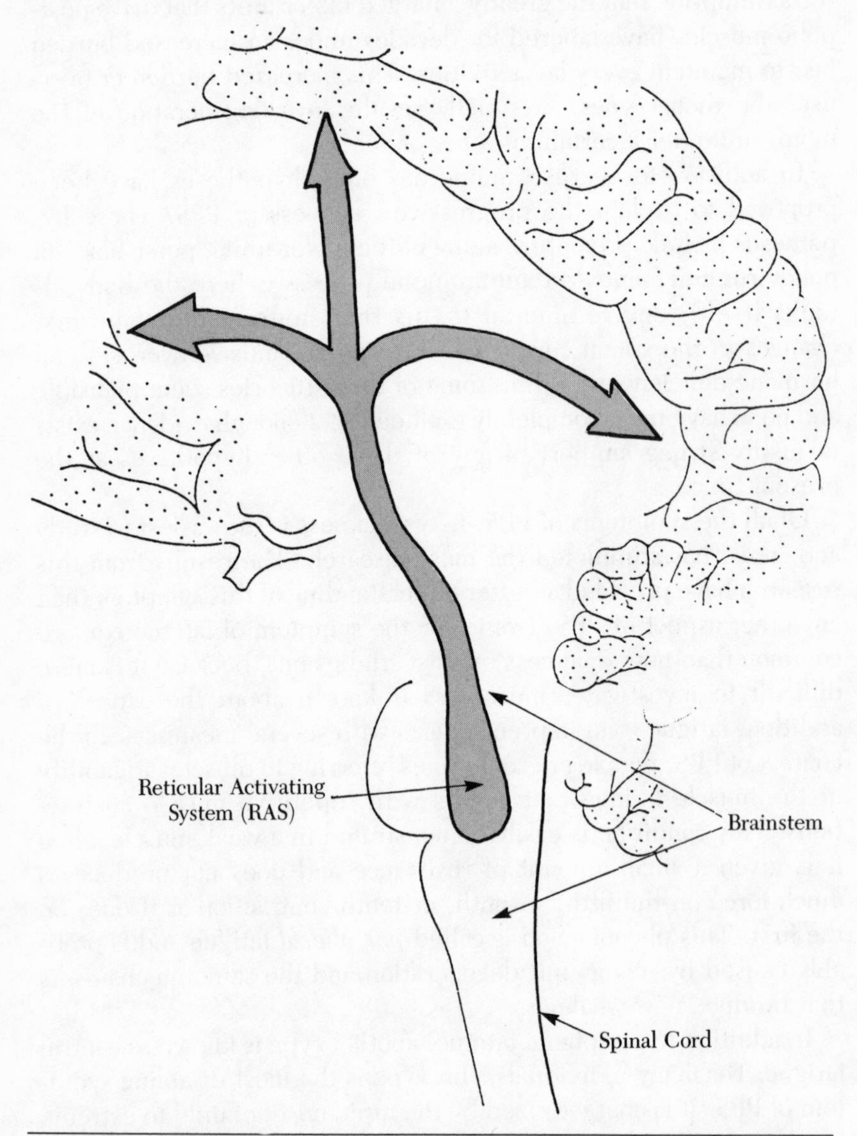

Legend: A cutaway side view of the brain and brainstem. The dark arrows represent specialized tracks of the ascending reticular activating system (RAS) which helps maintain wakefulness and mental alertness.

Another explanation for central fatigue locates the problem in the brain rather than in the motor unit. This theory suggests that central fatigue may be caused by abnormal function of a group of cells in the brain called the reticular activating system or RAS (Figure 1.5). These cells were often invaded and possibly damaged by the poliovirus during the acute illness. The cells in the RAS are responsible for maintaining wakefulness and mental alertness. Unlike the anterior horn cells in the spinal cord, which can be studied rather easily, there are no simple techniques to investigate the cells of the RAS directly. Much less is known, therefore, about their possible abnormal function.

To summarize our current understanding of the lifetime experience of polio, it is now clear that a fourth stage of poliomyelitis is experienced by approximately 20 percent to 40 percent of individuals who had paralytic polio many years ago. Typically, this fourth stage, called PPS, is associated with new weakness, generalized fatigue, and pain in muscles and joints. The new weakness occurs *only* in those muscles and nerves originally infected by the poliovirus and is believed to be caused by a degeneration or breakdown of affected motor units. The cause of generalized fatigue is less well understood.

2

New Health Problems in Persons with Polio

LAURO S. HALSTEAD

This chapter provides an overview of the evaluation and management of new health problems being experienced by persons who had paralytic polio years ago. The first section presents the criteria for diagnosing post-polio syndrome (PPS) and some of the basic issues that need to be considered in making the diagnosis. This is followed by a discussion of some of the risk factors or variables researchers have identified that are often associated with persons who develop PPS. Finally, there is a summary of the general strategy many clinicians use in approaching the evaluation and differential diagnosis of the post-polio individual. The second part of this chapter describes the evaluation and management of the six most common new health problems reported by polio survivors. In addition, there is a brief review of important issues to be considered by persons undergoing surgery and an overview of what is known about the prognosis of PPS.

MAKING A DIAGNOSIS OF POST-POLIO SYNDROME

The criteria for diagnosing PPS are listed in Table 2.1. New weakness is the cardinal symptom of PPS. Without a clear history of new weakness, the diagnosis cannot be made. In addition, the diagnosis of PPS cannot be made without excluding other likely causes of weakness. For this reason, PPS is called a *diagnosis by exclusion*.

Table 2.1 Criteria for the Diagnosis of Post-Polio Syndrome

1. A prior episode of paralytic polio confirmed by history, physical exam, and typical findings on electrodiagnostic exam.
2. Standard EMG evaluation demonstrates changes consistent with prior AHCD[1] (exam not required for limbs with obvious polio paralysis).
3. A period of neurologic recovery followed by an extended interval of neurologic and functional stability preceding the onset of new weakness; the interval of neurologic and functional stability usually lasts 15 or more years.
4. The gradual or abrupt onset of new weakness in polio-affected muscles; this weakness may or may not be accompanied by new health problems such as generalized fatigue, muscle atrophy, joint and muscle pain, decreased endurance and diminished function.
5. Exclusion of medical, orthopedic, and neurologic conditions that may be causing the health problems listed in number 4 above.

[1]AHCD = Anterior Horn Cell Disease

When making the diagnosis of PPS, several other considerations need to be kept in mind. First, symptoms such as pain and fatigue are fairly common and non-specific. Ruling out *all* possible causes, therefore, is not practical and can be prohibitively expensive; second, coexisting medical, orthopedic, and neurological conditions may be present and can produce very similar symptoms. Deciding which symptoms are caused by PPS and which symptoms are caused by another condition can be extremely challenging for even the most experienced clinician. As shown in Figure 2.1, once a problem such as weakness or pain occurs—regardless of the underlying cause—it may initiate a chain reaction of other complications that makes the original problem difficult or even impossible to identify. A common example occurs when new weakness (Figure 2.1, A) develops in the thigh muscle that supports the knee. The loss in strength may decrease the stability of the joint, leading to knee pain (Figure 2.1, B). To minimize the pain, the individual then uses that leg less frequently (Figure 2.1, C), which, in turn, leads to additional weakness and increased pain. If the cycle continues, the original problem of new weakness is often obscured by time and the pres-

Figure 2.1 Perpetuating Cycle of Symptoms

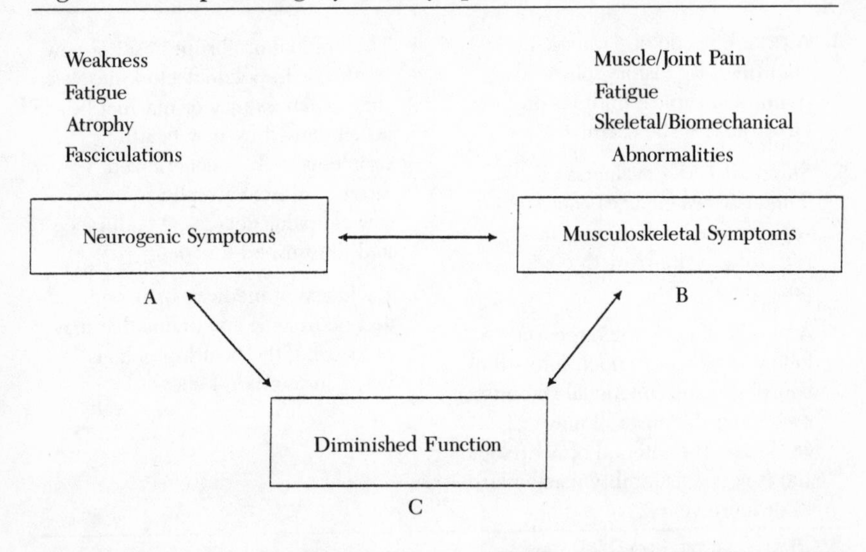

Legend: The onset of a symptom, e.g., weakness (A), may lead to the development of a second symptom, e.g., joint pain (B), which, in turn, may result in diminished function (C), which may then produce additional weakness.

ence of other symptoms. To clarify the initial symptom takes patience and persistence.

Risk Factors for Post-Polio Syndrome

A number of studies have found that the persons most at risk or most likely to develop PPS were those who experienced severe polio initially and, more particularly, those whose original losses were largely regained during the period of recovery. *It is not unusual, however, to see individuals with typical post-polio syndrome who had seemingly very mild acute polio followed by an excellent recovery.* Besides severity at onset, other risk factors identified in research studies include a greater length of time since onset of polio, the presence of permanent impairment following recovery, a recent increase of weight or physical activity, and being older at the time of diagnosis. One study also found that women are more likely to develop PPS than men. Most commonly, the onset of new problems is gradual, but in many persons, the outset may be triggered by specific events, such as a minor accident, a fall, a period of bed rest,

Table 2.2 Step-by-Step Approach to Evaluating Individuals with Possible Post-Polio Syndrome[1]

1. Confirm the original diagnosis of paralytic polio.
2. Determine the extent and severity of current deficits of strength, stamina, function, etc.
3. Develop a list of reasonable alternate explanations of each symptom.
4. Perform diagnostic tests to exclude or confirm non-PPS causes for each symptom.
5. If other causes diagnosed, treat and then assess need for remaining rehabilitation/medical interventions.
6. If no additional causes diagnosed, establish an objective baseline of function and a plan for rehabilitation/medical interventions.

[1]Adapted from the Post-Polio Task Force Recommendations (unpublished).

or surgery. Typically, individuals report that a similar event experienced several years earlier would not have caused the same decline in health and function.

Evaluation: General Principles

The evaluation of post-polio individuals with new health problems presents a challenge because of the general nature of many of the symptoms and the absence of special diagnostic tests. This challenge is further complicated by the continuing uncertainty of the underlying cause and the lack of any medications or treatments that might result in a cure. In light of these circumstances, it is important that even the most knowledgeable health professional follow a systematic, "step-by-step" approach to the evaluation of every individual who might have PPS. The steps are outlined in Table 2.2.

Confirming the original diagnosis of paralytic polio has to be based on the medical history and physical examination. If these are inconclusive, a standard electromyogram (EMG) should be performed. Old medical records are usually not available and, if they are, they can be unreliable for several reasons. First, there was often considerable pressure to make a "diagnosis" of polio to secure funding for hospitalization and treatment. Second, diagnostic facilities were not uniformly available to all individuals, especially those in lower socioeconomic groups and rural settings. Third, in the midst of an epidemic, there was a tendency to "lump" all persons who had even vague polio-like symptoms under the diagnostic label of polio.

If an individual was too young at the time of the illness to remember specific details and family or relatives are unable to provide additional information concerning the presence of weakness or paralysis, then a person's recollection has the same limitation as the old medical record. Particularly problematic are individuals who had nonparalytic polio, but because of the nature of the circumstances (e.g., they had painful muscles that made walking difficult for a time) they were told they had "paralytic" polio. Unless there are obvious signs on physical exam of characteristic muscle weakness and/or atrophy (muscle shrinkage), the only way to confirm a diagnosis of paralytic polio many years later is with an EMG exam.

Determining the extent and severity of current deficits uses the same diagnostic tools that were used in confirming a history of paralytic polio. Of particular importance is an assessment of how an individual functions throughout a typical 24-hour day and across the span of a week. The physical examination should emphasize a thorough neurologic evaluation and careful attention to muscle and skeletal abnormalities, such as scoliosis (spinal curvature), a difference in leg lengths, a decrease in range of motion in major joints and irregular patterns of walking. Deep tendon reflexes, such as the knee-jerk, are diminished proportional to muscle strength; sensation should be normal.

A limb that has been severely paralyzed may have *increased* sensitivity to light touch and pinprick; any *decrease* in sensation indicates some problem other than polio. For example, diminished sensation in one limb may suggest a radiculopathy (pinched nerve near the spine) or an entrapment neuropathy (pressure on an individual nerve such as that which occurs at the wrist producing carpal tunnel syndrome). Decreased sensation in all four limbs usually reflects the presence of a peripheral neuropathy (caused by a generalized disease of the peripheral nerves, such as diabetes). Increased reflexes suggest the presence of a disease process in the spinal cord or brain.

Because of the number, diversity, and complexity of the problems presented by many post-polio individuals, the staff at the National Rehabilitation Hospital (NRH) has found it beneficial to supplement, when appropriate, the standard medical history and physical exam performed by the physician with evaluations by other members of the rehabilitation team. Typically, this interdisciplinary team includes a nurse educator, physical and occupational therapists, and social worker or psychologist. Depending on the specific problems, an orthotist (bracemaker), respiratory therapist, dietitian or vocational counselor may also be involved. Referrals to pulmonologists, orthopedists, neurologists, and other specialists are made as needed. Of prime importance is the fact that, for many individuals, the evaluation in an established post-polio clinic is the first assessment done by a group of specialists who are knowledgeable and comfortable with polio and the features of PPS.

In addition to evaluations by members of the interdisciplinary team, the NRH staff recommend that most individuals obtain a standard electromyogram/nerve conduction study (EMG/NCS) of all four extremities and the paraspinal muscles (on either side of the spine) of the back and neck. The purpose of the EMG/NCS is to assess various aspects of the electrical activity of muscle and nerve function. This test is particularly helpful in evaluating limbs or muscles *thought* to be spared by the original infection but which, in fact, sustained subclinical (undetected) polio. The information obtained by these studies can also be helpful in prescribing appropriate exercise programs. In addition, this exam can provide clues that assist in diagnosing or excluding a number of other neuromuscular disorders. A summary of abnormalities found on EMG/NCS examinations in 108 subjects evaluated at the NRH Post-Polio Clinic in Washington, D.C., is listed in Table 2.3.

Based on the initial evaluation, a differential diagnosis or list of reasonable alternate explanations is developed for each of the major symptoms of PPS. Details regarding the differential diagnosis for each of these major symptoms are presented later in this chapter. As a rule, the NRH staff has not found it helpful to order a standard battery of screening tests for all individuals. Specific tests, such as a complete blood count (CBC), fasting blood sugar (FBS), creatine kinase (CK), thyroid function tests, etc., are obtained when indicated by the medical history and physical exam. Whether it is useful to monitor CK (a muscle enzyme) levels on a regular basis to assist in determining long-term prognosis or as an aid in clinical management is still not clear.

Table 2.3 Electrodiagnostic Findings in 108 Post-Polio Individuals

Findings	Percent
Carpal tunnel syndrome (CTS)	32
Ulnar neuropathy at the wrist[1]	2
CTS and ulnar neuropathy	3
Peripheral neuropathy[2]	3
Brachial plexopathy[3]	1
Tibial neuropathy	1
Radiculopathy[4]	4
Subclinical (undetected) polio	45

[1]Neuropathy: abnormality of one or more peripheral nerves.
[2]Peripheral neuropathy: abnormality of nerves in all four limbs (e.g., diabetic neuropathy).
[3]Brachial plexopathy: abnormality of a group of nerves that form the brachial plexus in the neck.
[4]Radiculopathy: abnormality of a nerve at its root or near where it exits the spinal cord.

Persons who had respiratory involvement initially and have a history of pulmonary disease, smoking, or scoliosis undergo a screening evaluation of their lung function with a forced vital capacity (FVC). If the FVC is less than 50 percent of the predicted value, additional tests of pulmonary function are obtained as discussed under respiratory complications later in this chapter. Individuals with significant spinal curvature are evaluated with a special scoliosis X-ray. If degenerative joint disease or DJD (wear-and-tear arthritis) or other skeletal abnormalities are suspected, X-rays of the appropriate joints are ordered.

To sum up, the assessments provided by special diagnostic testing are generally more fruitful in *excluding* certain conditions than assisting in the diagnosis or management of PPS. Despite the growing body of evidence suggesting motor unit deterioration as the cause of new weakness, there is still no objective method to predict who might develop PPS in the future or to monitor the progression of the underlying cause in those who are already becoming weaker. Specifically, no X-ray, blood test, or muscle biopsy, singly or in combination, can diagnose PPS. Instead, a careful, detailed clinical history must be relied on to distinguish between those individuals who have *no new weakness* (stable polio) and those who are experiencing *new weakness* (unstable polio) after a period of stability of at least 15 years. Finally, while elimination of all symptoms may not be possible, the NRH staff believes it is realistic to expect a large majority of those who come to the NRH Post-Polio Clinic to feel better both physically and emotionally and to achieve an improved level of function.

SPECIFIC HEALTH PROBLEMS

The major symptoms associated with PPS include new weakness, generalized fatigue, and pain in muscles and joints. The next sections in this chapter describe the evaluation, differential diagnosis, and management of these and other common health problems of polio survivors. The diagnostic strategies and therapeutic recommendations in these sections are based on the author's experience, the expertise of other clinicians, and studies in the medical literature.

Evaluation of Weakness

In a typical case of PPS, the presence of new weakness is determined by history. The new weakness is reflected in an individual's description of a decreased ability to perform specific tasks with the same ease or level of effort as in previous months or years. Weakness caused by PPS is often most prominent in those muscles that were severely involved in the initial illness and then underwent good recovery. Likewise, new weakness is commonly found in the so-called "good" limb that was felt to be spared but which, in fact, had subclinical polio and has been overworking for years to compensate for the more involved limb. By definition, polio-related weakness *does not occur* in muscles that were never affected by polio.

As a rule, diminished function tends to parallel muscle weakness. One of the characteristics of many polio survivors is their ability to appear normal or function at an extraordinarily high level of performance on relatively few good muscle groups. The random, scattered nature of the motor deficits and the body's uncanny ability to compensate with unconventional muscle and joint function make such performance possible. In this situation, late onset weakness of a single, critical muscle often disrupts a delicate balance that has been maintained for years. The disruption of this balance can result in a disproportionate loss of function that can be physically and psychologically devastating.

The physical examination of individuals with PPS weakness is helpful in documenting the absence of findings associated with other causes. The standard test for strength, the manual muscle test (MMT), is easy to perform and helpful in establishing a benchmark of strength; however, the MMT is of limited value for monitoring progressive weakness over time. Special equipment (e.g., Cybex, Cybex Corporation; Ronkonkoma, NY) is available to document precise, quantitative measures of strength and endurance, but this equipment is generally better suited for research studies and is impractical in most clinical settings.

The MMT evaluates the maximum strength of a single contraction, which can be surprisingly strong, even in a weakening muscle. However, the individual's history as to how his or her muscles function on a daily basis is more useful. Routine activities that require sustained or repetitive muscle contractions, such as walking, climbing stairs, or pushing a wheelchair provide a semiquantitative picture of declining strength. Current performance can be compared with similar activities in the past, e.g., number of stairs climbed or distance walked without difficulty one, three, or five years ago, versus the time of assessment.

Excluding other causes of new weakness in this population is absolutely essential. A list of common and not-so-common conditions that should be considered is summarized in Table 2.4. For most of these disorders, specific tests are available and an accurate diagnosis can usually be made. In searching for another cause of new weakness, it is important to remember that each one of the conditions listed in Table 2.4 can occur *in addition to PPS*. The most common and difficult diagnosis to exclude is *disuse weakness* (caused by decreased use of the muscle). As with PPS, disuse weakness can only be diagnosed through a careful history and ensuring that other neurological conditions are not present.

A person with PPS *weakness* often experiences a pattern of diminished strength, endurance, and function despite *no obvious change* in the usual level and intensity of activities. By contrast, a person with *disuse weakness* often describes a clear change—either gradually or abruptly—in the usual pace and intensity of physical activity or in the way that individual muscles are used. This change may occur when there is decreased activity because of pain or illness, a period of immobility, or a move to a less physically chal-

Table 2.4 Conditions That Cause Weakness

- Entrapment neuropathy (pressure on a peripheral nerve, e.g., median nerve at the wrist, ulnar nerve at the hand or elbow, peroneal nerve at the knee)
- Multiple sclerosis (degenerative disease of unknown cause)
- Myasthenia gravis (a neuromuscular disease treated with pyridostigmine, *Mestinon®*)
- Myopathies (diseases of muscles)
- Parkinson's disease (a degenerative disease of unknown cause)
- Peripheral neuropathy (disease of peripheral nerves, e.g., diabetic neuropathy)
- Radiculopathy (pinched nerve as it leaves the spine in neck or low back)
- Spinal stenosis (narrowing of spinal canal that compresses nerves in the neck or low back)
- Spinal tumors, abscesses, fractures, etc. (causing pressure on the spinal cord)
- Lou Gehrig's disease or amyotrophic lateral sclerosis (ALS)[1]
- Adult spinal muscular atrophy (a disease of unknown cause that attacks anterior horn cells)[2]

[1]Uncommon
[2]Rare

lenging home. Sometimes disuse weakness occurs when there is a shift in responsibility or a change in routine at work. Anything that produces *a more sedentary lifestyle* can result in disuse weakness. When disuse weakness is the most likely cause of diminished strength, a trial of carefully monitored exercise should be tried to determine if the new weakness can be reversed.

Management of Weakness: Bracing and Pacing

When new weakness occurs in muscles that have been consistently or maximally used in daily activities and the presumptive diagnosis is PPS, every effort should be made to provide more rest and support for those muscles. Examples include modifying activities and using adaptive equipment wherever possible, such as elevated seats, armrests, canes, braces, wheelchairs, or motorized scooters. It is worth noting that even simple adaptive devices (e.g., a cane) for ambulation have been shown to reduce energy expenditure significantly and occasionally reverse the loss in strength. In this way, seemingly small changes made throughout the day in both *what* an individual accomplishes and *how* various tasks are performed can produce an impressive change in the level of energy and sense of well-being.

In individuals who have been pushing themselves and their muscles to a maximum performance on a regular basis, a change in lifestyle with *more rest* and *less stress* is absolutely essential. Major lifestyle changes, such as switching jobs, retiring, or moving to a smaller, more accessible home, can be effective but are not always possible or practical. Changing priorities, eliminating nonessential activities, and creating rest breaks throughout the day are within everyone's reach.

Successful interventions must occur *at several levels*. It is not just an isolated muscle that needs rest but a way of life that must be modified. For this reason, when a new brace or crutch or modification of home is indicated, it should be prescribed together with a careful psychosocial assessment of the impact of recommended changes on family members, friends, and associates at work. Once new weakness is stabilized and a period of functioning without excessive effort or discomfort has been completed, then it is reasonable to explore the possibility of an exercise program.

Management of Weakness: Exercise

It is well known from muscle physiology that exercise of various types improves both muscle strength and endurance. Following episodes of acute paralytic polio in the past, individuals often went through long periods of exercise training and muscle re-education to regain the strength and muscle mass they had lost. In fact, exercise was frequently viewed as the "cure" for paralytic polio. The belief of many persons was that they could overcome or "beat" polio if they did enough exercises.

When people started getting new weakness many decades later, that same belief was still intact. As a result, many individuals resumed exercising on their own, often with a vengeance, frequently producing additional weakness. Based on these anecdotes and the initial theory that PPS was caused by overburdened motor neurons, it is understandable that most clinicians were cautious about prescribing any form of exercise. Now, more than a decade later, there is considerable evidence that almost everyone can benefit from some form of exercise. For many individuals, this level of exercise may be nothing more strenuous than gentle stretching or various types of yoga. For others, it may be considerably more vigorous and even include aerobic training. With this range of options, it is impossible to prescribe a set of exercises suitable for everyone. Instead, a list follows of general principles and guidelines that can be used by most people with PPS to develop a safe and effective exercise program:

- **Individualized and supervised program.** Exercise programs should be supervised initially by a physician or physical therapist experienced in neuromuscular diseases, if not polio. All programs should be customized to each person's needs, residual strengths, and symptom patterns. Given these constraints, research studies have shown that some polio survivors (but not all) can improve muscle strength (caused by new muscle hypertrophy and the growth of additional terminal axon sprouts) and enhance cardiovascular endurance with a closely monitored training program. In fact, some studies have reported an increase in strength in muscles both *with and without new weakness*.
- **Type of exercise.** There are numerous kinds of exercise. Finding the one that is right for each person and each limb often takes trial and error. Usually, it is a good idea to find two or more exercises that can be varied, exercising specific muscles every other day. For example, walking or exercising the lower extremities one day and alternating with an exercise for upper extremities the next day. This program provides a period of rest for each muscle group and variation that keeps the overall exercise program challenging and enjoyable. As a general rule, muscles that have a grade of 3 or less (using the muscle examination scale: 0 = no contraction up to 5 = normal strength) should be protected and not exercised; grade 3+ muscles can be exercised with caution; grade 4 and 4+ muscles can be exercised moderately; and grade 5 muscles can be exercised more vigorously.
- **Expect improvement.** Exercise should make one feel better physically or psychologically or both. If the activity is not strenuous enough to improve an individual's strength, much less the

cardiovascular system (e.g., stretching or yoga exercises), it still should give a psychological lift just to be doing a special activity for oneself on a regular basis.

- **Listen to your body.** Avoid pain, fatigue, and weakness. These symptoms are signals that your muscles have overworked. A brief period of fatigue and minor muscle pain for 15 minutes to 30 minutes after exercise is usually normal. Symptoms that last longer than 30 minutes to 60 minutes reflect muscle overwork and possible injury. If this occurs, the exercise should be reduced or stopped. *Any exercise that causes additional weakness should be discontinued immediately.*
- **Pacing.** Pacing has been shown to be safe and effective in increasing strength in some individuals. The intervals of exercising can be as short as two minutes to five minutes alternating with equal intervals of rest. The evidence also shows that secondary symptoms, such as generalized fatigue, can be reduced as individuals become conditioned and are able to perform more work with less expenditure of effort.
- **Use your best muscles.** Polio is often a focal, asymmetric disease with variable amounts of weakness in different limbs. Exercise the limbs least affected or those completely unaffected by polio, while avoiding the more affected extremities. For instance, if only the legs were affected, then the arms can be used in a fairly strenuous program that includes swimming or using an upper extremity arm bicycle; meanwhile, the legs will usually get adequate exercise in the course of doing daily activities.
- **Hydrotherapy.** Water therapy was the exercise of choice for many persons during their recovery from the original polio. It is still excellent therapy. Because of the buoyancy of water, it allows people to do things they can't perform on land. For especially weak limbs, inflatable cuffs can be used to float an extremity. For other limbs, water resistance provides a workout that can be fine-tuned to each person's strength. The principal disadvantages of hydrotherapy are that the temperature may not suit one's body and it may be difficult to find pools that have lifts (if needed). Also, the surfaces around pools tend to be slippery and dangerous for anyone with a tendency to fall.

- **Warm-up and cool-down.** As with other exercise programs, a warm-up followed by gentle stretching should be done to improve flexibility and reduce the possibility of injury. After exercising, a cool-down period should take place. Finally, the type of activity should be one that the participant enjoys to minimize the potential for dropping out because of lack of interest.

Evaluation of Fatigue

As mentioned in Chapter One, fatigue is a nonspecific complaint with a variety of possible causes. Adding to the confusion, people frequently use the same word to describe very different phenomena. For some, it means muscle fatigue or weakness, which is called *peripheral* fatigue in the scientific literature. For others, fatigue refers to a generalized sensation felt throughout the body. This is called *central* fatigue, which is discussed below.

Generalized fatigue is often described as overwhelming exhaustion with occasional flu-like aching and a marked change in the level of energy, endurance, and even mental alertness. Many people experience both this kind of central fatigue and peripheral fatigue (muscle weakness). In a study of polio survivors and healthy controls, each group described fatigue as "tiredness and lack of energy." Polio survivors, however, were significantly different from the control group in that they also described their fatigue as "increasing physical weakness," "increasing loss of strength during exercise," and "heavy sensation of the muscles."

Generalized fatigue usually occurs every day and tends to progress during the day. It is typically brought on by an accumulation of activities carried out previously on a daily basis without special effort or noticeable aftereffects. For many, it peaks by midafternoon or early evening, a phenomenon that feels to some like "hitting a wall." When this fatigue occurs, it is helpful for individuals to stop what they are doing, rest, and, if possible, take a short nap. Sometimes this is all it takes to reverse the fatigue and restore a sufficient sense of energy and well-being to continue through the remainder of the day without undue discomfort. Of all the new post-polio problems, generalized fatigue is often the most distressing and dis-

Table 2.5 Conditions That Cause Fatigue

- Anemia (low red blood cell count)
- Cancer
- Chronic alveolar hypoventilation (under ventilation of the lungs)
- Chronic infections
- Chronic systemic disease (diabetes, lupus, etc.)
- Depression
- Disrupted sleep
- Fibromyalgia (a condition causing fatigue and pain)
- Heart failure
- Hypoxemia (low blood oxygen)
- Medications
- Thyroid disease

abling; it is difficult to treat and imposes limits on people's lives without obvious physical changes that others can easily identify.

Before making a diagnosis of PPS fatigue, it is necessary to exclude other conditions that can cause this symptom (Table 2.5). Some of the more common disorders include anemia, depression, fibromyalgia (a musculoskeletal disorder that causes generalized muscle pain and fatigue), diabetes, thyroid disease, cancer, and autoimmune disorders (where the body attacks itself).

Fatigue occurring upon awakening usually reflects sleep disturbances that can be caused by a variety of conditions, including musculoskeletal pain, restless leg syndrome, or respiratory abnormalities. Fatigue that tends to last all day is not typical of PPS and may indicate chronic fatigue syndrome among other diagnoses. Depression can be associated with fatigue as can deconditioning, stress, and obesity. Prescription medications, such as beta blockers or sedatives and over-the-counter medications such as antihistamines, can contribute to feelings of fatigue as well.

Management of Fatigue

The management of fatigue follows many of the same principles as interventions for weakness and pain. Thus, improving one symptom will often result in an improvement in others. Knowing this should help individuals in their resolve to make significant changes in their lifestyles and priorities. It should also help physicians and other health professionals to provide persistent encouragement to make meaningful changes in daily routines, even if only one at a time.

Once other medical causes of fatigue have been ruled out, a careful evaluation of lifestyle is essential. Many people are more active and competitive than they realize: awakening early, working one job and sometimes two before coming home to more chores and demands, and then getting to sleep late. No matter what their vocation or avocation, many polios sustain a level of activity more strenuous than warranted by their strength and endurance. Often it is the equivalent of *running a marathon every day*. Not surprisingly, there is little or no reserve left by the end of the day or week. If this is the case, reducing energy expenditure by modifying one's lifestyle is the most important priority. A helpful way to think of this idea of "conservation of energy" is to imagine each day's supply of energy as a full tank of gas. Everyone has a fixed number of gallons to spend throughout the day. The goal is to be prudent in how each drop of gas is used so there is always some left at the end of the day.

Unfortunately, changing one's way of life is never easy. For polio survivors, it can be particularly difficult as many of them have worked hard to overcome their initial paralysis and have achieved a high level of performance and personal fulfillment. They may no longer perceive themselves as disabled and believe the long struggle to conquer polio is over, even if some visible impairment remains. Instead, new limitations unexpectedly and abruptly develop 30 years to 40 years later. People still expect, however, to regain lost function and feel better by persevering and working harder when they should follow the advice to slow down.

As a result, compliance with recommendations can be a significant problem. In one study, less than half of the subjects used a prescribed brace—and then only sporadically. Seventy percent refused to use a recommended crutch or cane simply because they didn't want to. In another study, the reasons stated for not following suggested interventions included: inability to change job or lifestyle, inability to lose weight, unwillingness to wear orthotic equipment, and inability to change jobs or purchase equipment for financial reasons. On the other hand, when subjects implemented one or more recommendations, they reported less fatigue and pain and an improved sense of well-being.

Despite obvious obstacles, many strategies are still available to help improve compliance, for example, having an old brace repaired rather than prescribing a new one. Another strategy is to begin with a small, more acceptable intervention that may help pave the way for a larger one later. People often reject anything that publicly advertises their disabled status. Changes that enable them to retain some sense of control may enhance compliance, such as displaying a handicapped placard in the windshield instead of going directly to handicapped license plates. Someone who has been ambulatory for 35 years may reject buying a wheelchair but agree to try a cane or use a wheelchair in the airport. In time, the wheelchair may become more acceptable as the person realizes the cane is helpful but insufficient to relieve symptoms.

For many individuals, making changes means letting go of a routine that worked for years and changing behaviors that people believe are integral to their concept of self. Typical excuses include: "I never wore a brace," "I never needed a cane," "What will people say if I have handicapped plates?" and "My boss will think I'm *really sick* if I ask for a rest break." Countless variations on these themes have been heard over the years as people try to come to terms with their new limitations. What is gratifying is how many of the same individuals come back a few weeks or months later exclaiming, "Why didn't I make these changes years ago?," "My fatigue is better," and "The pain in my leg is gone."

Getting help through peer support groups is another way of coping with new disabilities. Support groups provide a mechanism for sharing advice and practical tips on how to improve independence and deal with the common obstacles of daily life. Hearing what someone else did to solve a similar problem is often far more persuasive than anything a health professional can say.

In addition to lifestyle changes and energy conservation techniques, preliminary reports suggest several medications that may be helpful in relieving PPS fatigue, including pyridostigmine (Mestinon®), amitriptyline (Elavil®), selegiline (Eldepryl®), and bromocriptine (Parlodel®). The most promising of these is pyridostigmine. In one study, researchers reported significant improvement in some measures of strength and a reduction in fatigue using 60-mg pyridostigmine three times a day. In a second evaluation of the same medication with the same dosage, investigators found almost 60 percent of subjects experienced a reduction in fatigue. Encouraged by this experience, researchers at the Montreal Neurological Institute and Hospital carried out a third study of pyridostigmine involving 126 persons. In this investigation, neither the subjects nor the researchers knew who was given real medicine and who received the placebo (a double-blind study). The results were reported in late 1997 and failed to show any significant improvement in either the strength or fatigue of subjects in the treatment group compared with those in the control group. Although these conclusions were disappointing, further research using pyridostigmine appears to be warranted.

In conclusion, the successful management of both new weakness and fatigue is essentially accomplished through a succession of small changes rather than by one dramatic intervention. Occasionally, there is a "magic bullet" and a single recommendation will produce a startling improvement in symptoms. However, that is the exception, not the rule. More commonly, an improved sense of well-being arrives, little by little, after a series of small steps. The important thing to remember, especially in the beginning when the symptoms are overwhelming, is that each small change adds to the others and together they eventually provide significant relief. With time and persistence, most people *do* feel better. For example, walking with a cane may improve the symptoms by 15 percent; installing elevated seats at home may contribute another 10 percent; a mid-day rest may add another 15 percent or 20 percent; shopping only once a week or by phone may relieve the symptoms by an additional 15 percent; and losing five pounds may add another 10 percent of improvement. No single change by itself would be very impressive. But taken together, this set of five interventions might provide as much as 65 percent or 70 percent improvement to an overall feeling of well-being.

Evaluation of Pain

Pain of muscles and joints is the first or second most common symptom in the majority of clinical studies of individuals with PPS. The number of disorders that cause pain is extensive, but an assessment should begin with conditions commonly associated with chronic musculoskeletal wear and tear and disorders that have significant muscle and/or joint manifestations. Table 2.6 lists the more common conditions that should be excluded.

Table 2.6 Conditions That Cause Pain

- Bursitis (inflammation of the lining of joints)
- Fibromyalgia (a condition causing muscle fatigue and pain)
- Myofascial pain (pain of muscle and connective tissue)
- Osteoarthritis (also called degenerative joint disease)
- Polymyalgia rheumatica (a disease affecting muscles and joints)
- Polymyositis (a disease causing inflammation of muscles)
- Rheumatoid arthritis (a chronic disease that affects primarily joints)
- Tendinitis (inflammation of tendons)

Many of the problems that appear to be related to *overuse* of weak muscles and abnormal joint movements may simply represent the inevitable consequences of any chronic disability. There is no evidence that these problems are any more common in polio survivors than they are in individuals with other muscle and joint diseases. To facilitate the diagnosis and treatment of pain, we developed a classification at the NRH clinic that divides the different kinds of pain into three categories.

Type I pain or *post-polio muscle pain* (PPMP) is felt only in muscles affected by polio. It can occur both as a *superficial burning* discomfort or as a *deep muscle ache*; many polios say the latter pain is similar to the discomfort experienced during their acute illness years earlier. The deep pain is often characterized by muscle cramps, while the superficial pain is sometimes associated with fasciculations (involuntary muscle contractions or twitching), a crawling sensation, or extreme sensitivity to touch.

Type I pains typically occur when the individual tries to relax at night or the end of the day—often hours or even a day or two after the muscles were used. This muscular pain is frequently made worse by physical activity, stress, and cold temperature, and is alleviated with dry or moist heat, slow stretching, and rest. Definitive treatment usually requires bracing, crutches, or some other means of supporting and protecting weakened muscles.

Type II pain or *overuse pain* includes injuries to the soft tissue, muscle, tendons, and bursa (tissues surrounding a joint). Common examples are rotator cuff (shoulder) tendinitis, deltoid bursitis (in the shoulder region), fibromyalgia and myofascial pain (especially in muscles of the upper back, shoulders and neck). Myofascial pain (*myo*, muscle, *fascia*, connective tissue) in post-polio individuals is similar to that in other persons and is characterized by bands of tight muscles and focal *trigger points* that elicit a "jump" response when palpated. These pains are caused by poor posture or improper body biomechanics. Fibromyalgia is associated with fatigue and generalized muscle pain lasting three months or more with 11 or more of 18 specific tender muscle points. In one study, slightly more than ten percent of individuals evaluated for pain in a post-polio clinic met the criteria for fibromyalgia and another ten percent had borderline fibromyalgia.

Type III pain or *biomechanical pain* presents as degenerative joint disease (DJD), low back pain, and pain from pinched nerves. The location of this pain is often related to the type of locomotion and individual use. Persons who are walking tend to have pain in the legs and low back, while individuals who use wheelchairs or rely heavily on crutches are more likely to have pain in the arms and hands. Weakness of polio-affected muscles and poor body mechanics accelerate the development of DJD as years of ambulating on unstable joints increase the energy expenditure to perform a given task. These costs accumulate silently until they cross a critical threshold.

In addition to back and joint complaints, symptoms related to nerve abnormalities are commonly seen in Type III pain. Typical examples include compression of the median nerve at the wrist or carpal tunnel syndrome (CTS), ulnar nerve impingement at the wrist or elbow, and cervical or lumbosacral radiculopathies (pinched nerves as they exit the spinal canal in the neck or low back). These conditions can cause pain and sensory loss *as well as weakness*. Persons who have used assistive devices, such as canes, crutches, or wheelchairs, are more likely to develop nerve compression at the wrist. As one would expect, the chances of this occurrence increase the longer the devices are used. Fortunately, these nerve injuries can be detected with EMG/NCS studies even before an individual has symptoms. Preventive measures can then be taken to minimize further damage.

A review of the records of 40 individuals evaluated consecutively in the NRH clinic revealed that almost everyone was experiencing one or more kinds of pain. The most common was Type III pain (biomechanical) and was diagnosed in three out of four persons. Slightly less than 50 percent of the group had Type II pain (overuse), and approximately 20 percent had Type I pain (post-polio muscle pain).

Joint pains are not typically accompanied by significant swelling, inflammation, or tenderness. X-rays of painful, weight-bearing joints show degenerative changes proportional to the amount of stress the joints have sustained. Even in seriously deformed joints, with the possible exception of the joints in the spinal column, extreme degenerative changes are uncommon. Other diseases, such as rheumatoid arthritis, which involve the joints, may also be present. Their occurrence in post-polio individuals, however, is similar to the general population and, if suspected, appropriate X-rays and laboratory tests should be obtained.

Management of Pain

Successful pain management depends on the underlying causes and is based on a few principles supplemented by type-specific recommendations. These principles are: (1) to improve abnormal body mechanics, such as poor posture and gait deviations; (2) to support weakened muscles and joints; and (3) to promote lifestyle changes that conserve energy and reduce stress.

Using these principles together with specific recommendations, it is possible to reduce or eliminate the vast majority of pain symptoms. This expectation is leavened with two warnings. First, the individual must be willing and able to make the recommended changes. Second, permanent relief is usually difficult to accomplish as the continued stress and strain of daily activities tend to cause flare-ups of old symptoms and the onset of new ones.

Treatment for Type I pain (muscle) includes periodic rest, stretching, and heat together with assistive devices, such as braces and crutches; lifestyle modifications; and, occasionally, the use of medications. Passive and active stretching helps to relieve muscle cramping and tightness and maintain the flexibility of muscle and connective tissue. Stretching, when properly used, can provide surprisingly effective relief for this type of pain. However, it must be performed judiciously as there are situations when stretching tight, contracted joints can paradoxically compromise a person's function. A good example is a tight Achilles tendon in the back of the ankle, which can compensate for weak or absent calf muscles. In this instance, the tight tendon provides assistance in the "push-off" phase of walking. If it is stretched back to its "normal" length, the person will develop a limp on that side of the body and experience a significant increase in the "work" of walking.

A variety of medications have been used to treat PPMP, but the most common ones such as aspirin, ibuprofen (found under a variety of brand names including Motrin® and Advil®), acetaminophen (Tylenol®), and narcotics are of little use. For some persons, low doses of muscle relaxants, such as diazepam (Valium®) or lorazepam (Ativan®), taken at bedtime can provide good pain relief. However, the dosage may need to be adjusted to provide nighttime rest while avoiding daytime fatigue or impaired concentration. Some individuals have also obtained good relief with low doses of antidepressants such as amitriptyline (Elavil®) used at bedtime or fluoxetine (Prozac®) taken in the morning. Although both of these medications are primarily antidepressants, they are often used to treat pain resulting from other causes besides PPS. An added benefit of treating PPMP with medications taken at bedtime is the observation that individuals frequently become less fatigued, possibly because of improved sleep.

Treatment for Type II pain (overuse) incorporates many of the same principles and specific recommendations used in managing Type I pain. When overuse leads to soft tissue injuries of tendons, ligaments, and bursa, anti-inflammatory medications like ibuprofen can be invaluable and occasionally even provide long relief. These medications, however, must be used judiciously as they have the potential to cause serious side effects, such as stomach ulcers and kidney damage. Less dangerous is superficial heat (in the form of hot packs) or deep heat (such as ultrasound) which can be used as primary therapies or as supplements to other interventions.

Heat is effective because it relieves muscle spasms, increases blood flow, improves the elasticity of the soft tissues, and promotes healing of local inflammation. Subjectively, it provides sedation and relaxation, reduces the perception of pain, and decreases joint stiffness. Cold in the form of ice packs is also effective and has the advantage of providing longer lasting relief than heat. Another alternative to medications is TENS, which uses a painless electric current applied to the skin to block pain fibers. When there is a severe injury to a tendon, such as that which occurs with rotator cuff tendinitis (frozen shoulder), steroid injections or even surgery may be indicated. However, in most cases, the best treatment is attempting to rest the affected area by protecting the joint and decreasing overuse.

Treatment for myofascial pain begins by relieving any aggravating factors such as poor posture and abnormal gait. The next step is a trial of myofascial relief techniques, including "spray and stretch" with a cooling agent such as ethyl chloride, and trigger point injections with a local numbing agent such as lidocaine. Physical therapy treatment using massage, stretching and local heat is also effective.

Treatment for Type III pain (biomechanical) is directed at improving posture and back care together with decreased weight-bearing and stress on unstable joints. Abnormal biomechanics can often be modified with fairly simple and practical interventions that affect repetitive activities, such as sitting, standing, walking, and sleeping. Common examples include a lumbosacral (low back) cushion used in the car, office, and favorite chair at home to support and rest back muscles; a shoe lift that helps equalize a leg length discrepancy; and a "buttock lift" (small portable pad) placed under an atrophied (shrunken) hip muscle that levels the pelvis while sitting. Individuals should select chairs that do not tilt, have a firm, padded seat, a back that extends to the shoulder blades and padded armrests that support elbows and shoulders. During sleep, a firm mattress—cushioned with a two inch or four inch foam "egg-crate" mattress—provides a measure of softness on top with good underlying support.

When persons with carpal tunnel syndrome must use a cane or crutch, special handles known as *pistol* grips are helpful. These handles have a broad surface area that can be rotated to maintain the wrist in a neutral position and increase the weight-bearing surface of the palm. The goal is to minimize further damage to the median nerve in the wrist.

For genu recurvatum (back-kneeing) resulting from quadriceps' weakness or genu valgus (knock-knee) caused by ligamentous instability, a long leg brace or knee-ankle-foot-orthosis (KAFO) with a free ankle joint and an extension stop at the knee may be helpful. Those with ankle dorsiflexor weakness (muscles that lift the foot up) or ankle instability may benefit from a short leg brace or ankle foot orthosis (AFO), high-top shoes, or even cowboy boots fitted with zippers to make them easier to put on.

In a study of lower extremity braces prescribed in one post-polio clinic, orthotics were recommended for the following reasons: to improve safety by reducing the risk of falls, to reduce pain, and to decrease fatigue by improving gait efficiency and symmetry. Subjects who used orthoses reported significant improvements in pain relief, especially at the knee. Despite the new plastics and lightweight metals used in making braces, they are often discarded. Sometimes the braces are not cosmetically acceptable. Frequently, individuals prefer to repair and use their old, familiar braces than to start over again with new ones, which may disrupt their muscle "substitution" patterns and create a new set of problems. Sometimes people simply resist using any kind of braces at all for psychological reasons.

Although most types of polio pain may be temporarily relieved by the interventions described above, definitive treatment usually requires major interventions that affect one's lifestyle: new bracing, crutches, a motorized scooter, less walking, less work, less pushing—whatever it takes to provide permanent support and protection of weakened, tired muscles. For some individuals, complete rest may not be possible because they have to rely on affected joints or limbs for locomotion, self-care, and activities at home or work. In these instances, there is no easy answer. The physician must work with the person's family and friends as well as marshal whatever support services are available in the community, such as the Visiting Nurses Association, Meals-on-Wheels and volunteer groups.

In summary, unlike many other pain syndromes, the pain of PPS should respond fairly promptly to appropriate interventions. Muscles that ache because of weakness and overuse feel better and can even become pain-free, if the principles of bracing and pacing are applied consistently. Joints that hurt because of excess weight-bearing, poor posture, or abnormal biomechanics do improve, and often dramatically, with rest, proper support, and better alignment. The real challenge is how to remain pain-free throughout an active day. Finally, pain that persists during periods of rest, diminished stress, and with adequate support of the spine and joints is almost always caused by something other than PPS.

Evaluation of Respiratory Complications

During the acute phase of polio, the most feared complication was impaired respiratory function. Approximately 15 percent of persons with paralysis during the epidemic years of the late 1940s and early

1950s required the use of an iron lung. Many years later, these same individuals have the greatest risk for developing new pulmonary problems. In one study of persons successfully weaned off a respirator after their acute illness, almost 40 percent required ventilatory assistance on a full- or part-time basis many years later.

Another group likely to experience new respiratory complications are those who developed severe scoliosis (spinal curvature) in the years following their initial paralysis. Other pulmonary problems seen among polio survivors include obstructive lung disease (usually from smoking cigarettes or chronic asthma), restrictive lung disease (RLD) from chest muscle weakness, and chronic alveolar hypoventilation or CAH (under-ventilation of the small air sacs in the lungs caused primarily by weak breathing muscles). Additionally, some individuals develop sleep-disordered breathing. In a study of the frequency of symptoms suggesting sleep-disordered breathing, researchers found the most common complaints were waking frequently, followed by snoring and fatigue. These findings were significantly different from a nonpolio comparison group.

RLD is one of the most common disorders among persons with a history of respiratory involvement. In this condition, the lungs and rib cage do not expand normally because of weakness of the muscles that control respiratory inspiration (chiefly, the diaphragm and chest wall muscles). This weakness can be aggravated by obesity, scoliosis, smoking, asthma, or other lung diseases.

An evaluation of persons with complaints of respiratory difficulties begins with questions concerning any previous need for respiratory support, the length of time such support was required, the use of tobacco, and any history of other pulmonary diseases, including chest infections. The examiner should also ask about snoring or nighttime awakening, daytime sleepiness, headaches (especially in the morning), shortness of breath, and impaired cognition. During the examination, special note should be made on inspiration and forced expiration of wheezes, evidence of obstructive lung disease, as well as for the presence and degree of scoliosis.

Persons with a history of respiratory difficulties, or those who are at risk of developing pulmonary complications, should have their vital capacity or VC measured (both sitting and lying down), along with their maximum inspiratory and expiratory pressures and maximum ventilatory volume (MVV). The MVV measures the maximum amount of air that can be breathed in and out rapidly in 12 seconds. This test is especially useful in polio survivors as it reveals if the muscles of breathing are likely to fatigue when there is a respiratory complication. Individuals who have difficulty bringing up mucus from their lungs should also be evaluated for their maximum insufflation capacity (maximum volume of air-stacked breaths) and assisted and unassisted peak cough flow.

In addition to these studies, another test commonly performed to evaluate lung function is the arterial blood gas (ABG). This measures, among other things, the amount of oxygen (O_2) and carbon dioxide (CO_2) in the blood. When a sleep disorder is suspected, overnight blood O_2 and CO_2 saturation monitoring is desirable. Recent investigations have shown that even if these results are normal, a sleep study is necessary to clarify the nature and severity of sleep disturbances.

Management of Respiratory Complications

The evaluation and management of individuals with respiratory complications must be under the care of a pulmonologist, a physician specializing in pulmonary medicine. Whenever possible, it is preferable to have a pulmonologist who is knowledgeable in the management of persons with neuromuscular diseases such as polio or muscle disorders such as muscular dystrophy. Such knowledge is necessary because the complications that occur and interventions used in polio survivors can be quite different from those used in individuals with normal muscles and nerves.

With this in mind, the following comments are meant solely as a brief overview of some of the more important points regarding the management of respiratory complications in post-polio individuals. The recommendations are in no way intended to serve as a substitute for being closely followed and monitored by a competent pulmonologist.

The symptoms of sleep-disordered breathing, RLD and CAH can usually be improved with inspiratory positive pressure, which can be delivered in several ways. Continuous positive airway pressure (CPAP) or bilevel positive airway pressure (Bi-PAP), which independently varies inspiratory and expiratory pressures, is used to manage sleep-disordered breathing. Pressure or volume-regulated portable ventilators and Bi-PAP at higher inspiratory pressures (15–30 cm H_2O) are used to treat RLD and CAH. These therapies can be delivered via an oral, nasal, or oral-nasal mask. Because of the development of newer noninvasive methods of delivering positive pressure, a tracheostomy is seldom needed and should be avoided if at all possible.

Negative pressure body ventilators (NPBVs), such as the iron lung, the Porta-lung, and the chest shell, are still options for some individuals. Drawbacks to these devices include sleep interference, poor portability, and a high occurrence of apnea (interrupted breathing), hypoxia (low blood O_2), and hypercapnia (high blood CO_2). Other ventilators that work directly on the body are the intermittent abdominal pressure ventilator and the rocking bed. These have some of the difficulties of NPBVs and are generally less effective.

Frog breathing or glossopharyngeal breathing (GPB) is a method of using the tongue and pharyngeal muscles to project a "gulp" of air past the vocal cords into the lungs. Immediate vocal cord closure traps the air in the lungs. This technique is not difficult to learn but has not been widely used since the last big epidemics of the 1950s. In a study of individuals trained in GPB, slightly more than half used it while speaking to keep a more consistent volume and duration of sound despite a mechanical ventilator; approximately 20 percent used it when changing mechanical breathing aids; and the remainder did not practice or use the technique at all. People who become expert at GPB can take up to 200 cc of air per "gulp" and, with repetition, can achieve almost 3 liters per "breath."

Additional considerations for persons with impaired lung function include the use of assisted coughing (beginning with the lungs as full of air as possible) to help clear airway secretions when the muscles of expiration (mostly the abdominal muscles) are weak. Mechanically assisted coughing (with a small machine) is more efficient and less labor-intensive than manual techniques. Either manual or mechanical chest percussion can help with atelectasis (lung collapse) or mobilization of secretions. All persons with impaired pulmonary function or a history of recurrent respiratory infections should receive influenza vaccines each year in the fall and the Pneumovax vaccine (for pneumococcal pneumonia) every ten years.

Evaluation of Swallowing Problems

Along with respiratory failure, dysphagia or difficulty in swallowing is one of the most dangerous complications of acute polio. Dysphagia occurs when the virus damages nerves that supply muscles of chewing and swallowing. These nerves are located in the brainstem or bulbar region of the brain which is located just above the spinal cord. Persons whose polio involves these nerves are said to have *bulbar* polio.

During the big epidemics in the past, severe dysphagia was fairly uncommon, occurring only in 10 percent to 15 percent of those who developed paralysis. In studies of PPS, the number of persons reporting new swallowing problems is about the same. However, the degree of severity varies greatly from mild complaints of food and pills sticking in the throat to problems with choking, gagging, and even aspiration pneumonia (caused by food or fluids going down the "wrong tube" into the lungs).

Evaluation of dysphagia includes a modified barium swallow (MBS) as well as pulmonary function tests. The MBS is a special video X-ray performed while the individual swallows foods of varying properties, such as crackers, paste, and liquid mixed with barium (an X-ray contrast material). Persons with a history of difficulty in swallowing during acute polio are much more likely to have an abnormal MBS test or new swallowing problems than those with no prior history of dysphagia. However, several studies have shown swallowing abnormalities in persons who had *no swallowing problems* either at the time of the study or during their acute illness with polio. These findings suggest that there was subclinical (undetected) involvement of the bulbar nerves with the original viral infection.

The differential diagnosis of dysphagia includes structural abnormalities from the mouth to the stomach as well as any disease or injury that involves the muscles of swallowing. One must bear in mind that a second cause of dysphagia may coexist with polio.

Management of Swallowing Problems

Management of dysphagia should be under the care of a professional who diagnoses and treats this disorder on a regular basis. Speech and language pathologists frequently have special expertise in this area and swallowing disorder clinics are often found in larger medical centers.

Recommendations that can improve swallowing include the following:

- Change the consistency of the food or liquid to substances that go down more easily
- Turn the head to one side
- Tuck the chin
- Alternate food and liquid
- Avoid eating when fatigued
- Eat smaller and more frequent meals
- Never swallow with the head and neck thrown back in extension or while talking or laughing.

Swallowing difficulties appear to remain stable in the majority of persons with dysphagia. However, progression of symptoms does occur, so periodic reevaluation is recommended.

Evaluation of Cold Intolerance

Many polio survivors experience difficulty in tolerating cool or cold temperatures. Sometimes they have more trouble than others keeping a limb or even the whole body warm in winter, despite the amount of clothing used. At other times, they have an unpleasant sensation of cold in one or more limbs, even in a warm room or in warm weather.

Cold intolerance is also associated with other sensations and changes. For example, individuals may experience color changes in the skin ranging from reddish blue to violet to blanching (whitening) of an affected extremity, as well as flushing and the sensation of hot and cold flashes. These sensations and changes can be accompanied by an increased sensitivity of the skin, a burning-type pain, and decreased manual dexterity. These symptoms may be caused by a combination of factors including: (1) reduced blood flow through areas of small, atrophic muscles; (2) a malfunction of sympathetic nerves (part of the autonomic nervous system damaged by the polio virus at the time of the original infection) that normally regulate the flow of blood in and out of limbs; and (3) reduced muscle contractions that allow cooled blood to pool and contribute to swelling in the limbs. These factors produce increased sensitivity of specialized receptors in the vessels, resulting in further arterial narrowing and reduced flow of warm blood to the extremities.

On examination, the core body temperature is almost always normal but limbs with significant atrophy (muscle shrinkage) tend to be cool to the touch with a bluish discoloration and variable amounts of swelling. The strength of the pulse is usually directly related to the amount of atrophy in that extremity unless other diseases are also present.

The history of cold intolerance and findings on exam may be altered by a number of other medical conditions, such as anemia, decreased thyroid function, peripheral neuropathy (from diabetes, for example), congestive heart failure, and peripheral vascular disease. Proper diagnosis and treatment of these disorders may significantly improve the symptoms of cold intolerance caused by PPS.

Management of Cold Intolerance

The management of cold intolerance is largely symptomatic. Multiple layers of clothes are useful, especially when placed on the affected extremities first and then on the rest of the body. Massages (always toward the heart) and short-term use of local heat (20 minutes or less) are also effective. Special care must be taken by any person using heat who has a diagnosis of peripheral vascular disease or diminished sensation in a limb. To avoid burns, the source of heat should always be in contact with normal skin as well as the area being treated. The heat source should be padded and laid on top of the person or affected limb. Paradoxically, heat applied to the abdomen can also make the extremities warmer through a reflex mechanism. Some people report relief with the use of nylon panty hose and woolen long underwear, even in warm weather, when air-conditioning creates sustained cool interiors and unexpected drafts of cold air.

Surgical Considerations

There are many types of surgical procedures and many reasons for individuals to have surgery. The medical literature contains numerous anecdotes—both positive and negative—about surgical experiences in polio survivors. However, there are very few studies about the effects of surgery or anesthesia in post-polio individuals and no rules can be applied to everyone. The decision to have surgery is a personal one. The best advice is to make the decision with care and with as much information as can be obtained.

If the effects of polio are minimal and surgery is going to be performed under local or regional anesthesia (only a part of the body is numbed), then no special precautions are necessary other than the same ones observed with any minor surgery. On the other hand, for someone with significant polio involvement—either in the past or present—who is going to have surgery that requires general anesthesia or GA (the individual is completely asleep), then it is imperative to consult a pulmonologist (lung doctor) and an anesthesiologist (anesthesia physician) before scheduling surgery. These two specialists, together with the surgeon and yourself, must work together as a team. The persons at greatest risk of complications during GA are those with a history of ventilatory use or swallowing difficulties; persons with involvement of the shoulders, arms, or trunk; and individuals with a history of respiratory problems, such as smoking, asthma, repeated lung infections, or significant scoliosis (curvature of the spine).

The surgeon, pulmonologist and anesthesiologist should all be familiar with the details of an individual's polio history and with any respiratory problems or special needs, such as positioning, required during surgery. In preparation for surgery, the pulmonologist should obtain lung function tests beforehand and be available following surgery to monitor progress closely. Likewise, the anesthesiologist should review the different types of anesthesia and muscle relaxants that are available and select the ones best suited for each person's particular needs. For individuals undergoing GA, another issue to discuss with the anesthesiologist concerns whether to use an endotracheal tube or a laryngeal mask airway. Persons with a history of disorders of the stomach and esophagus (the tube which carries food to the stomach) have an increased risk of aspiration (stomach contents coming up into the lungs). To prevent aspiration, it is preferable to use an endotracheal tube (a tube inserted into the upper part of the lungs) than a laryngeal mask airway.

Table 2.7 Important Considerations When Getting Ready For Surgery

- Talk with someone (preferably a person with polio) who has had a similar surgical procedure. If you cannot find someone in your area, try to locate someone on one of the post-polio bulletin boards on the Internet.
- Be aware that minor surgery on a totally paralyzed limb can result in delayed healing because of decreased blood supply.
- Elective surgery is always preferable and allows you time to get in as good physical shape as possible. This may include losing weight, stopping smoking, starting an exercise program, etc.
- Operating rooms are cool. If cold intolerance is a problem, notify the surgeon and anesthesiologist to provide extra padding and blankets to maintain adequate warmth. Also ask about forced air warmers. These are fairly new devices which are available in most operating rooms and are designed to keep you "toasty" during surgery.
- Invite a family member or a friend to join you during your visits to the pulmonologist and anesthesiologist so someone else will be familiar with your concerns. This person can be your advocate during surgery and while you are recovering from anesthesia.
- If you have a choice, select the hospital that has had the most experience with post-polio individuals or other neuromuscular conditions.

If in pursuing answers to these and other concerns, individuals do not feel they are being heard or are not getting the attention they want, it is imperative to seek a second opinion. There is no occasion in living with PPS when an individual needs to be more assertive and better informed than at the time of a surgery that requires GA. See Tables 2.7–2.9 for additional considerations.

Prognosis

No studies exist that predict life expectancy for polio survivors. Nor are there any data about the frequency of common life-threatening conditions, such as heart disease, cancer, and stroke. PPS is most directly life-threatening when there are pulmonary complications or severe swallowing difficulties.

Table 2.8 Important Considerations During Surgery

- Anesthesia and muscle relaxants are designed to decrease nerve and muscle function. If there are fewer nerve and muscle cells because of polio, then the normal amount of these medications may be excessive. The dosages, therefore, need to be carefully adjusted to meet the altered requirements of each individual.
- In general, "polio" muscles tend to be more sensitive to muscle relaxants than normal muscles. Anesthesiologists experienced with polio survivors having surgery recommend using about half the normal dose of muscle relaxant or even less. To make this judgment more scientific and help assure a safe dose, your response to muscle relaxants can be measured during surgery using a special device called a nerve stimulator.
- If muscle paralysis is prolonged, a ventilator is used to breathe for the individual until he or she can breathe independently. This is standard procedure. With careful monitoring, usually no problems occur.
- Regional anesthesia is usually preferable, if this is an option, because it involves fewer drugs and tends to have fewer side effects. A recent study reports that a widely used medication, lidocaine, may cause nerve damage when used for spinal anesthesia (medication inserted through a needle into the space around the spinal cord). If this finding is confirmed, other anesthetic drugs (e.g., bupivicaine or tetracaine) could be used instead.
- Local or regional anesthesia is often supplemented with a sedative given through the veins. The purpose is to improve the individual's comfort. However, this sedative can create additional problems such as aggravating sleep apnea. Whenever possible, persons should try to avoid this type of sedation; if it is given, they should anticipate a delay in their recovery.

Several studies have found that the chances of developing heart disease and stroke may be increased in some individuals because of the presence of certain risk factors, such as increased weight, elevated cholesterol, and a sedentary lifestyle. In most persons, as in the rest of the population, these risk factors are amenable to change. However, these changes never come easily for anyone, especially with the combination of excess weight and reduced mobility. Many people find it helpful to seek the advice of a nutritionist while others can only lose weight in a group setting, such as Weight Watchers or special weight-loss clinics sponsored by local hospitals.

Table 2.9 Important Considerations After Surgery

- Close monitoring of pulmonary function is critical, especially after general anesthesia. Lung function is worse for everyone for the first 48 hours after surgery.
- Sleep apnea may become worse following an operation with general anesthesia.
- Polio-affected muscles may be temporarily weakened after general anesthesia, which, in turn, may increase the need for ambulatory support or the use of other aids and devices.
- Depending on the person's age, extent of paralysis, and length of surgery, recovery from surgery may be prolonged two, three, or more times beyond what is expected for others. (E.g., recovery that normally takes 2 weeks may require 4 weeks to 6 weeks or more).
- A diet high in protein is generally desirable following surgery to help tissues heal more rapidly.
- Request a supervised program of graded exercises to help reverse the effects of bedrest, pain, reduced function, etc.

As far as muscle strength and function are concerned, the new weakness of PPS appears to be a slowly progressive benign process for the great majority of persons. One study found an average loss of strength of one percent per year in subjects studied for an average of just over eight years. Other studies have found little or no change in strength in persons followed for five years or more. While these are very reassuring findings, they clearly do not reflect the experience of all individuals with PPS. Post-polio clinics across the country still track many thousands of persons who have had dramatic losses in strength and function and who, despite all interventions, continue to lose strength each year.

For the majority of persons who find the new symptoms of PPS overwhelming, however, there is good news. With persistence and common sense, most of the symptoms of PPS can be improved with a combination of lifestyle changes, "bracing and pacing," and medications. In addition, a significant increase in the amount of research being done in this country and abroad in recent years offers the hope of a better understanding of the cause of PPS and more effective treatments.

3

Aging, Comorbidities, and Secondary Disabilities in Polio Survivors

JULIE K. SILVER

Aging, comorbidities, and secondary disabilities can all profoundly impact persons with polio and post-polio syndrome (PPS). Understanding these factors and their effects will help polio survivors in functioning at their highest levels.

AGING WITH POLIO

Strength decreases gradually as everyone ages. In most people, this change in strength is so subtle that it is almost imperceptible from year to year. In persons who have had polio, however, the loss of strength through *normal aging* may not be so subtle. Persons who have had polio have fewer energy reserves and are often functioning at a maximal level; therefore, even a small change in strength may herald a more noticeable change in function. For example, the effort required by a person with polio who walks with crutches and braces may tax whatever strength they have. If they then lose a portion of their strength, even if it is only a small amount, it may be enough to keep them from walking. The change from walking to not walking is a big loss in terms of function, which came about from a small loss in strength.

Probably the most accepted theory with respect to the cause of PPS is the concept of increasing muscular weakness due to overuse. Muscles that lost part of their nerve supply because of the initial polio are now supplied by surviving nerve cells. These cells are really doing two jobs: supplying the muscles they were initially intended to supply and supplying muscles that lost their original nerve supply. Years of trying to perform double duty has led to a growing vulnerability of these nerves which actually begin to malfunction much sooner than expected.

Overuse combined with normal aging can cause profound changes in strength. Unfortunately, time marches on and nothing can be done about the normal loss of strength caused by aging. The loss of strength because of overuse can be dramatically improved, however, through increased awareness and appropriate medical intervention. The concept of "use it or lose it" departs from the reality faced by polio survivors. In fact, polio survivors' motto should be more along the lines of "overuse it and you will lose it"! Polio survivors must test their mettle as they age and meet the challenges of growing old with polio, armed with the knowledge and determination to maintain the highest possible level of function.

COMORBIDITIES

Comorbidities are illnesses or medical conditions (other than polio) that may impact one's overall health and/or ability to function. Common comorbidities include diabetes, heart disease, arthritis, high blood pressure, thyroid problems, and cancer.

Comorbidities may significantly impact a polio survivor's ability to perform at his or her usual level. For instance, a polio survivor who also has heart disease may be experiencing symptoms of fatigue. This fatigue may be caused by either the heart disease or the post-polio syndrome, or it may be a combination of both conditions. Whenever there is more than one diagnosis, it is important to consider how each condition might be contributing to a polio survivor's symptoms.

SECONDARY DISABILITIES

Secondary disabilities occur when persons disabled by a particular injury or illness become further disabled because of a second injury or illness. For example, a polio survivor who uses a short leg brace but does not require any assistive devices (e.g., crutches) might become further disabled by a fall causing a hip fracture. In this case, the person may now need the short leg brace and a cane and may be unable to walk as far as he or she could before the fall. The secondary disability is not the fall or hip fracture; rather, the secondary disability is the increased difficulty in walking. By contrast, the fall is the event that caused the disability, and the hip fracture is the injury or impairment. Another example might be a polio survivor who sustains an injury to his or her rotator cuff (that is, the group of muscles and tendons in the shoulder that allow overhead activities) and now is unable to style his or her hair. The secondary disability is the *new difficulty required to do something.* In this case, styling the hair becomes more difficult or even impossible, thus resulting in a secondary disability.

Sometimes secondary disabilities persist despite treatment of the inciting injury or illness. For example, in the case of the person who sustained a hip fracture, the fracture will certainly heal with appropriate treatment; however, the person may be unable to walk as easily as he or she did before the fracture and may always need to use a cane for stability. In other cases, where an underlying injury such as a rotator cuff tear goes undetected, seeking appropriate medical treatment may cure the injury and eliminate the secondary disability.

The Importance of Comorbidities and Secondary Disabilities

Both comorbidities and secondary disabilities may cause someone to lose the ability to function in their usual capacity. Because polio survivors are often functioning at a maximal level without many energy reserves, even a small change in their health status may result in an inability to continue to perform at their usual level. One may think of this scenario as a delicate balancing act where even a subtle shift may cause a pronounced effect.

The good news is that many, if not most, medical conditions can be effectively treated by experienced health care providers. Therefore, seeking early treatment of new symptoms can help minimize the effects of comorbidities and secondary disabilities on polio survivors.

The Relationship of Osteoporosis, Falls, and Secondary Disabilities

Osteopenia is a term used to denote bones that are thin and fragile. Osteoporosis technically means the bones are thin and fragile and that a fracture has occurred with less than the usual amount of force required to break a healthy bone (called a pathologic fracture). However, since the terms osteopenia and osteoporosis are commonly used interchangeably, the term osteoporosis will be exclusively used throughout this section.

Paralyzed limbs almost certainly have osteoporosis because strong muscles are required to keep bones strong and thick by pulling on them routinely. A lack of muscle tension is almost always associated with bones that are thinner than normal. In bones that are very thin, a fracture may occur with or without trauma. The most common fractures occur in the hip bones, vertebral (spinal) bones, and bones in the forearm. Vertebral fractures often occur without any history of trauma and are found only after someone complains of back pain. Fractures in the arms frequently occur when individuals stumble and try to break their fall with their hands. Hip fractures are also commonly associated with falls and frequently cause secondary disabilities. Recovering from a hip fracture is often difficult, even in the best of circumstances; however, in the case of polio survivors, it can be daunting.

Persons with polio are certainly not destined to suffer the ill effects of osteoporosis and the consequences of falls. While osteoporosis in a paralyzed limb is difficult (if not impossible) to treat, preventing osteoporosis in other bones is important. Women should consult with their primary care physicians before menopause and discuss hormone replacement therapy. Men should also consult their doctors about ways to prevent bone loss as they age. Recent studies of new medications have been very encouraging; such medications *may even reverse some of the bone loss that has already occurred.*

Falls are a major cause of injury and disability in persons who are polio survivors. For some individuals, falling has become a way of life. In fact, falls may have occurred so often that an individual considers himself or herself an *expert* in the art of falling. Therefore, many people who have had polio underestimate the risks associated with falling and do not take enough precautions to avoid falling.

Often people ask, "How many falls are too many"? The answer is that even one fall is too many if that fall happens to cause serious injury. Keep in mind that even a gentle fall can result in an injury and subsequent disability, especially if there is significant bone loss or osteoporosis.

4

How to Find Expert Medical Care

JULIE K. SILVER

The old adage, "The mind doesn't know what the eyes haven't seen," certainly applies to doctors confronted with caring for persons who have had polio. Persons with polio often correctly comment, "My doctor doesn't know how to treat polio patients." Because acute poliomyelitis had essentially been eradicated (by vaccinating children) when today's physicians were in training, few physicians had the opportunity to become familiar with the disease. Consequently, most doctors who are practicing today have never seen a case of acute poliomyelitis. Additionally, while many physicians currently care for individuals who have a history of old polio, they do not necessarily have a great deal of experience in treating problems related to the initial polio or the symptoms of post-polio syndrome (PPS). To make matters worse, many of the symptoms of PPS may be subtle or may mimic other common medical conditions. A physician who has not had the opportunity to evaluate many people with old polio may not be skilled at diagnosing and treating someone with PPS.

Fortunately, there are physicians and other health professionals who have a special interest in treating polio-related problems and have developed an expertise in this field. Finding these experts may feel like looking for a needle in a haystack; however, as PPS becomes more widely reported and understood by the medical community, health-care providers are gradually becoming more interested and knowledgeable about polio and PPS. While accessing "state-of-the-art" medical care may still be challenging, the following guidelines will hopefully make the process easier.

STEP 1: CHOOSING A PHYSICIAN

In today's complex medical environment, everyone needs someone directing his or her medical care. This task is generally that of the treating physician who is responsible for making an appropriate diagnosis and then generating a treatment plan based on the diagnosis. Choosing a physician who has expertise in treating polio-related problems is the first step in obtaining appropriate medical care.

Understanding the roles of different physicians is critical in finding the right doctor. The following is a list of physicians by specialty and a summary of how they may participate in the care of persons who have had polio. This list is not meant to be exhaustive; certainly, many other types of specialist physicians may be valuable to consult.

Primary Care Physicians

Primary care physicians (PCPs) have generally had additional training after medical school in one of two areas: internal medicine or family practice. Therefore, they are often referred to as internists or family practitioners. As a rule, PCPs monitor all ongoing medical problems and counsel people on preventing many medical conditions. When a medical issue is complicated or out of their area of expertise, they commonly refer the individual to a specialist for counseling and treatment. Finding a good PCP is worthwhile, regardless of whether one has had polio. Think of the PCP as the quarterback on a football team. He or she will "call the plays." A PCP who is thoughtful, knowledgeable, and thorough is ideal. If he or she is not an expert in polio-related problems, then appropriate referrals should be made to medical professionals who have the expertise. Even if the person is referred elsewhere, the PCP remains the quarterback and should be kept informed of any treatment plans, such as changes in medications as this may affect other medications and/or medical conditions.

Physiatrists

Physiatrists are medical doctors who have spent at least four years after medical school training in Physical Medicine and Rehabilitation. The specialty of physiatry actually evolved in part as a response to the need to care for injured World War II veterans and to care for individuals during the polio epidemics in the early to mid-1900s. Dr. Robert L. Bennett, who was chairman of the American Board of Physical Medicine and Rehabilitation from 1953–1963, stated, "I am convinced that it was through contact with patients who had polio that physiatrists first were established as clinicians with the special interest, essential training, and recognized competence to handle those conditions that required carefully prescribed activity." Once called physical therapy doctors, physiatrists today are experts in prescribing exercise, but their expertise extends far beyond this definition. Most physiatrists have had extensive training in treating polio-related problems, and many physiatrists routinely treat people with a past history of polio. Not surprisingly, many of the prestigious polio clinics in the United States are directed by physiatrists.

Neurologists

Neurologists spend at least four years after medical school specializing in the field of neurology. Neurologists have treated polio throughout history and, like physiatrists, are specialists in treating PPS. Both neurologists and physiatrists are excellent at caring for individuals with polio; however, generally only one of these specialists is involved at a time. This situation is simply because most people do not need both a neurologist and physiatrist (both of whom would perform similar functions) treating them simultaneously for polio-related problems.

Orthopedists

Orthopedists (also called orthopedic surgeons) have at least five years of training after medical school in orthopedic surgery. Generally, orthopedists do not coordinate the care of persons with polio, but rather than intervene when there is a specific orthopedic or musculoskeletal problem. While orthopedists are experts in surgery for these problems, they also may be involved in nonsurgical treatment. Not all orthopedists, however, have experience in treating persons with a history of polio. Therefore, persons considering surgery should inquire about their surgeon's experience.

Ideally, someone who has had polio in the past will have a good relationship with a PCP who may or may not have expertise in polio-related problems. If the PCP is not an expert, then the person should be followed by a physiatrist or neurologist who has a special interest in polio and PPS. These polio survivors should also be referred to an orthopedist when appropriate. Some PCPs are experts at treating respiratory conditions and others may prefer to defer to a pulmonologist.

Rarely does an expert in polio-related problems rely solely on his or her own skills without referring to appropriate specialist physicians, therapists, orthotists (brace makers), etc. Because a team of experts is ideal, many centers have been set up across the country with specialty polio clinics that integrate all of these experts in the care of persons with polio.

STEP 2: FINDING A PHYSICIAN

As noted above, ideally a good PCP will be able to direct someone who has had polio to appropriate specialists; however, not all situations are ideal and sometimes even good PCPs are not aware of the various resources and the medical professionals in their area who may have expertise in polio. Motivated by the need to find medical caregivers with expertise in treating polio-related problems, polio survivors have banded together and formed nearly 300 support groups nationally. One of the primary goals of these groups is to disseminate information on the latest medical breakthroughs in PPS. Another important goal is to relay information regarding where polio survivors can be evaluated and treated by medical personnel who specialize in treating PPS (see Appendix for a list of resources).

STEP 3: BEFORE THE FIRST VISIT

Before going to an expert in polio, consider the following:

- Will my insurance cover the cost of this treatment?
- If not, can I afford to pay the balance?
- Is the building/office accessible?

Table 4.1 Information to Give to Your Doctor

1. Current problems or symptoms listed in order of importance.
2. Brief history of initial polio (age at onset, length of hospitalization, etc.).
3. Other medical illnesses or injuries with the respective dates (e.g., diagnosed with diabetes—1987, left hip fracture after a fall—1994).
4. Past surgeries, including dates.
5. Current medications.
6. Allergies to medications.

- Is this a one-time visit or will I have follow-up appointments?
- How urgent are my problems? Can I afford to wait for the next available appointment?

Although these questions may seem obvious, many people fail to consider them prior to seeking medical care. Certainly, addressing these issues in advance will prevent unwanted surprises (such as a big bill after the visit).

STEP 4: GETTING THE MOST OUT OF THE OFFICE VISIT

Preparing for a visit to the doctor can be valuable for both the patient and the physician. All physicians have a set schedule. Although physicians notoriously run late, there is increasing pressure for them to stick to their schedules. Anything a polio survivor can do to make the visit more efficient will benefit both the patient and the treating physician. In medical school, physicians are taught to obtain information from a patient in an orderly and distinct manner. Coming prepared with a printed copy of this information will allow the treating physician to spend much less time on "housekeeping details" and focus more time on specific problems and complaints. Table 4.1 is an example of what information should be included. Bringing any old medical records, X-rays, reports, etc. may also be helpful. Notes from initial polio hospitalizations are generally not useful; however, they may be included if readily available.

Knowing in advance how much time the doctor spends on a new evaluation is helpful. Also, knowing whether this is a one-time evaluation or whether there will be follow-up appointments can be important. Regardless of how much time the physician has allotted, it is important to be clear and concise. The temptation to reminisce and explain the acute poliomyelitis in great detail should be avoided simply because of time constraints. Instead, focus on whatever issues are current and provide pertinent information at the specialist's request. A focused patient in turn helps the physician focus on relevant and important medical issues and presents the opportunity to explore treatment options in greater detail. Finally, be realistic with expectations for the visit. Doctors are seldom miracle workers. Persons with realistic expectations will generally find the help they need.

STEP 5: WHAT TO EXPECT FROM AN EXPERT

During the visit, the doctor will take an oral history (which should be supplemented with written notes from the person seeking treatment as described above) and perform a physical examination. Extensive manual muscle testing is often not done by the physician, but may be done by a physical therapist. Often a gait analysis is done as well as a review of all assistive devices (e.g., canes, crutches, etc.) and orthotics (braces).

Once the physician has reviewed all of the pertinent data and performed a physical examination, he or she will make appropriate recommendations. These recommendations may include blood tests, an electromyogram (EMG), X-rays or other imaging studies such as a magnetic resonance imaging test (MRI), physical, occupational or speech therapy, new braces or refurbished old ones, and a wheelchair or scooter evaluation. Finding appropriate medical care may be frustrating for some polio survivors; however, a systematic and organized approach will make the process much easier and the likelihood of success much greater.

5

Energy Conservation

GRACE R. YOUNG

Polio survivors have a history of overcoming enormous personal obstacles. For those dealing with the late effects of polio, it can seem disheartening to realize that fatigue comes more quickly, and formerly successful lifestyles must be modified. Coping with post-polio syndrome requires some choices. By understanding the neurological basis of polio's late effects, respecting the body's requirements for activity and rest, and minimizing physical stress, life can still be full and enjoyable if lived with strategy and vision.

USING YOUR BODY EFFICIENTLY

A lot has been written about body mechanics, and the basic principles of good body mechanics. There are no rigid rules that apply to all of us, especially since polio survivors have individual patterns of muscle weakness and unique ways of compensating.

Good posture uses much less energy than "slumping." It helps prevent muscle tension, fatigue, backaches, and neck pain. It even enhances appearance which helps your attitude and self-confidence. The muscles in your body work to keep you upright against gravity. With your head up, trunk straight, and shoulders back, your body balances itself on its own bony framework so the muscles have less work to do.

Sitting decreases the demand on the cardiovascular system and relieves the weight bearing joints of the lower extremities. Sit during meal preparation and cleanup, while working on hobbies out in the garage, and while showering and dressing. When shaving, applying makeup or styling your hair, sit down and use a prop-up mirror on the counter. Sit while gardening. If you analyze and plan, almost any activity can be accomplished while sitting.

Lifting and unlifting (setting the load down) are potentially hazardous. Improper movements can squander energy and cause back injuries. Before starting to lift, assess the situation. Where is the load located in relation to your waist? How much does it weigh? Must it be carried and how far?

It seems as if most materials that need to be lifted are located below waist level or on the floor. The solution is to lift from a sitting position. First estimate the weight by pushing the load with your foot, crutch or cane. If it does not push easily it is too heavy for you to lift safely even if sitting, so ask for assistance. If it feels okay, sit close and lift the load onto your lap, then place it on a shelf or table. Do not get out of the chair while holding the load.

To lower loads that are located above your shoulders, test the weight first by pushing up on it. Keep the load as close to your body as possible and let it slide down onto your lap if you are sitting or onto a table, cart or counter if you are standing. Do not lift heavy items over your head; ask for assistance.

The principles to remember are: (1) test the weight of the load; (2) keep it close to the body; (3) have a surface ready to receive it.

Carrying objects changes your center of gravity and can stress your shoulders and arms and overuse your leg muscles. This is one area where a few changes can save a lot of energy. Use mechanical help for carrying. There are several pieces of inexpensive equipment which I consider front-line necessities in the effort to conserve energy. These include:

- A kitchen utility cart on casters, available in most houseware departments, can be your best ally. Just one trip with the cart will transport the dishes, glasses, silverware, and food from the counter to the table and back again. Keep frequently used condiments and seasonings on a tray on the bottom shelf of the cart, ready to put on the table. Use a cart to carry laundry or cleaning items. Push it along when you straighten the house. Consider placing two or three carts in strategic locations throughout the home; many more uses will come to mind.
- A lightweight luggage cart and a collapsible wheeled grocery cart are useful for many things besides traveling. Take them to

the mall to carry purchases. Use them for transporting articles from room to room and between the car, house, or office. If your house is multi-level, use them to carry objects up and down steps. Keep the carts open and in a central location, ready to use anytime.

Protecting Your Joints

Let's begin with the advantages of using wheelchairs and motorized carts, especially if you use a cane, Lofstrand crutches, or underarm crutches. Long-term use of crutches or canes can cause secondary complications such as nerve compression in the neck area (thoracic outlet syndrome) or wrist (carpal tunnel syndrome) which can cause pain, numbness, tingling and even weakness in the arm and hand. In addition, continuous use over many years of walking aids can cause gradual weakening of shoulder and arm muscles, even if these areas did not appear to be affected during the initial attack. Some muscles may have suffered subclinical damage, in that motor neurons were lost during the acute attack but not enough motor neurons to be obvious during normal daily usage. Heavy use of canes or crutches over a long period of time can overwork the remaining motor units. And, last but not least, ambulating uses a tremendous amount of energy when you have weak legs.

Manual Wheelchair, Electric Wheelchair or Motorized Scooter

With strong arms, good trunk stability and no pain in your upper extremities, a manual wheelchair may fill your needs. It folds and transports easily in an ordinary car. But this is not a level world. Rough terrain and inclines will challenge the strength of upper extremities, placing them at risk for pain and new weakness.

Choosing between a motorized scooter or electric wheelchair can be difficult. Wheelchairs require a full-size van with a lift, while electric lifts for scooters can be installed in a minivan, station wagon or pickup truck. A scooter, however, requires the ability to transfer on and off easily, as well as a certain amount of trunk and upper arm strength and upper body balance. If these areas are already experiencing new weakness, it might be more economical in the long run to purchase an electric wheelchair now.

The advantage of having mobility with little energy expenditure far outweighs the initial expenses, and many insurance companies cover durable medical equipment (DME) when it is prescribed by a physician.

External Support to Protect or Compensate for Weak Joints

When a joint is surrounded by weak muscles or when an imbalance between weak and strong muscles exists, it can cause increased stress on the ligaments, causing them to stretch. It then takes more work and therefore more energy to stabilize a wobbly joint. This results in increased wear and tear which can lead to degenerative arthritis, deformity, and pain. Once joints are damaged, they will not be able to regain their original function.

Along with wheelchairs, nothing conjures up as much dread as the idea of having to start wearing braces or splints. However, external support to compensate for weakness frequently offers so much relief from pain and joint instability that your energy level and sense of well-being are enhanced. Here are a few examples:

- When the quadriceps muscle at the front of the knee is too weak to support the weight of the body during ambulation, the knee may hyperextend ("back knee") so that the ligaments instead of the muscles are providing much of the support during weight bearing. Problems like these lead to gradual deterioration of the knee joint. A long leg brace (Knee, Ankle, Foot Orthosis or KAFO) can keep the knee joint from shifting during ambulation.
- Weak muscles at the front of the ankle can cause a "foot drop," where you cannot bring your foot upward so your heel hits the ground first. To keep from stubbing your toe and possibly falling, your leg has to lift higher to clear the floor. In this case, a short leg brace (Ankle, Foot Orthosis or AFO) supports the foot and ankle in proper alignment, allowing the heel to strike the ground first.
- When one leg is shorter than the other, your center of gravity changes with each step. This is fatiguing unless the discrep-

ancy in leg length is compensated by a lift, either inside or outside the shoe.

- Weakness in the wrist or thumb muscles can cause the arm to compensate by moving in ways which quickly fatigue the whole upper extremity, including the elbow and shoulder muscles. Hand or thumb splints place these joints in a functional position.

Prevent Pressure on the Thumb Side of Your Fingers

Often when we lift or carry objects, we use our hands in a manner that pushes the fingers away from the thumbs. This can cause deformities at the knuckles, with the fingers eventually angling away from the thumb ("ulnar drift"). Here are some ways to avoid this problem:

- Carry objects such as a purse on your forearm and not with your fingers. When carrying casserole dishes, wear oven mitts and place your palms under the dish instead of lifting with your fingers. Use two hands for lifting pots and pans. Wear oven mitts and grip the pot handle with one hand, palm down, while the other hand holds the side of the pot.
- When drinking from a cup or mug, place both hands around the vessel. Lifting a cup of liquid by the handle pushes the fingers into ulnar drift. Use two hands for pouring from half-gallon milk or juice containers.
- Do not carry garments on clothes hangers with your fingers. Fold the garments over your forearm for carrying. Push doors closed with your palm, not the thumb side of your fingers. Car door openers enable you to use pressure from the palm, not the fingers, to push the handle in or upwards.

Use the Largest Joints Available for any Activity

Joints closest to the trunk are the largest and strongest. Shoulders, elbows, and hips are more stable than wrists, fingers, and feet. Carry heavy objects such as books, notebooks, packages, dishes, etc., with your palms up and the weight of the object distributed between your palms and forearms. This puts the stress on the elbows instead of having the fingers and wrists carrying the whole load. For long distance carrying, use mechanical help.

Change Positions Frequently

Holding muscles and joints in one position for prolonged periods of time causes muscles to fatigue, placing more stress on the joints. Try not to hold onto objects for prolonged periods of time. Change positions every fifteen minutes or so, and when you are not using an object, put it down.

Use a typewriter or computer instead of writing by hand. For card players, a plastic or wooden card rack eliminates the need to grasp a fistful of cards. Book holders free your hands from prolonged gripping. If reading in bed is your style, there is a Bed Reader which allows you to read while reclining.

Using a telephone is a challenge if you have a weak arm. A head receiver set relieves one hand from having to keep a grip on the receiver while the other hand dials and writes messages. Some people use a telephone holder, but this doesn't furnish much privacy. Most local phone companies furnish headsets and other adaptive telephone equipment free of charge to individuals with disabilities.

Rest, Pacing and Timing

Rest is restorative. That sounds obvious, but remember that you are asking your body to carry out activities with weakened muscles. With normal muscles, motor units trade off with each other during muscle contractions, some units contracting while others are resting. In weakened polio muscles, the motor units are fewer in number and cannot trade off. They have to contract for longer periods and have less time to rest.

Muscle fatigue and pain must be respected. Muscle pain is a warning signal that the muscles have been overused and are in danger of suffering further damage, which is not always obvious while it is occurring. Listen to your body. Rest at least one hour during the day. Split the time into segments if you prefer. Employed people usually cannot rest at lunchtime, so it may be better to take a one-hour rest immediately after work. Afternoon rests make your evening activities more productive and enjoyable.

Pacing is important. We all have days when we feel so good that we take on an ambitious project and keep pushing hard so we do not lose momentum. Persons with post-polio syndrome must be particularly cautious, since we can be incapacitated for two or three days afterward. It is tempting to overdo on your good days. Overall, however, we can be more productive if we plan ahead and pace our activities.

"Day-at-a-Glance" and "Week-at-a-Glance" books are ideal for designing a schedule which will treat your body gently. Prolonged activities such as housecleaning, cooking or gardening need to be broken up into short segments with rest breaks in between. Use the "Day" book each morning to plan your work and rest periods. Decide on the time you will begin each activity and how long you will work at it, allowing 15 minute rest breaks every 30 minutes. Use a kitchen timer as a reminder.

When first starting this experiment, write down in the book how you feel when you finish each activity. "Tired," "muscles hurt," "feel better than usual," etc. This is important; it reveals whether your rest and pacing techniques are helping you accomplish the goals you are setting for yourself.

The "Week" book will help you alternate light and heavy activity days throughout the week. Split your ambitious projects into daily segments throughout the week and stick to the plan, no matter how good you feel on any particular day.

Timing can make a difference in how you feel. You may have different levels of pain and fatigue at various times of the day. Activities which are simple to perform in the morning may be very difficult later in the day. For example, if cooking supper in the late afternoon is stressful, prepare most of it in the morning, to be reheated later.

Filling in your "Day" and "Week" books may seem like a chore at first, but it will pay dividends in the future by helping to set priorities. People have told me that these books made them aware for the first time of the amount of stress caused by their daily activities.

An activity is too stressful if:

- There is a feeling of fatigue. This may seem obvious, but most of us have learned not to pay attention to our bodies. We were

all taught to ignore pain and fatigue and just keep on going. The level of fatigue may be out of proportion to the level of activity, but listen to your body. The activity may be too stressful, even if your mind says it should not be.
- There is a change in the quality of movement. Notice your motions when performing the activity. Is there a tremor or jerkiness?
- There is a change in the quantity of movement; that is, decreased range of motion. For example, you can usually lift your arm to a certain height but find that the height lessens as you continue the activity.
- You start to use compensatory movements. For example, you "hunch" your shoulder in order to raise your arm, or you swing your leg out to the side instead of flexing the hip while walking.

If any of the above signs occur while you are in the middle of an activity, it is time to stop and rest or modify what you are doing.

Eliminating and Delegating Jobs

When your energy level is limited, you need to think about your priorities. If you want to do the interesting and fun things or remain employed, you may have to reconsider the importance of excellence in housekeeping. It's hard to have it both ways when you have a chronic condition.

If making your bed is important to you, try using a lightweight comforter in place of both blanket and bedspread. You can make the bed before you get out of it. Pull up the top sheet and comforter while you are still in bed, then give a tug or two to straighten them after you get up.

Ironing is another big energy-user. However, manufacturers have given us a choice to iron or not to iron. Many dresses, blouses, slacks, even some linen items have enough no-iron synthetic threads in them that all you have to do is pull the garments out of the dryer while slightly damp, smooth them and hang them. If, on the other hand, ironing is a domestic ritual that you enjoy, lower the height of the ironing board and do it sitting down.

The second hardest modification to achieve is delegating jobs to other people. When you have worked hard to achieve independence and have done certain activities yourself for many years, it may seem like a step backward to ask others to do them for you. But remember, this isn't something that happens just to people with disabilities. When nondisabled people age, they lose some of their independence and have to ask for assistance. Those of us who have a chronic condition just reach this point a little sooner. If at all possible, hire someone to do your heavy housework.

When asking for help from family members, it is important to separate the necessary from the nonessential tasks. People offer their help out of love and respect and they may not do things exactly your way. You need to be flexible and show your appreciation.

You may be able to barter services with friends or neighbors. If you have bookkeeping or office skills or can sit with a new baby or older child, you can offer to trade your talents with someone who can do household chores. State employment offices and college or church bulletin boards are sources for hiring help.

CREATING A USER-FRIENDLY ENVIRONMENT

Few of us are lucky enough to be able to build a fully accessible house or to remodel our existing homes. Most of us have to live with what we've got. So we need to modify our surroundings to make them as energy-efficient as possible without incurring large costs.

Home Modifications

Adaptations can be as easy as substituting silk flowers for live plants, changing the location of objects, and organizing supplies. The following ideas are simple, inexpensive, and doable. They are designed to stimulate your thinking and help you create other ways to make your surroundings more user-friendly.

Correct Work Heights Preserve Energy

Remember the suggestion to sit whenever possible? Good advice, but counter-productive unless you pay close attention to the height of your work surfaces. You will not conserve energy if you rest your legs but exhaust your shoulder muscles because the work surface for your activity is too high. A work height is right for you if it allows you to keep your head up and back straight and is about an inch below elbow level. Here are some ideas for creating work stations at the proper height:

- Purchase a drafting chair at a discount or office supply store. The swivel seat adjusts with a pneumatic handle from 22 inches to 32 inches off the floor. The five-caster base is stable and rolls easily. Other features which are important for good body positioning: a footrest and an adjustable backrest. The one disadvantage is that the seat cannot be raised while you are sitting on it. Use caution to keep the stool from rolling while you lift yourself onto the raised seat. To play it safe, back the drafting chair against the bottom corner cupboards while getting onto it. Be sure to try this out at the store before you purchase this item.
- Create lower work stations by placing a large wooden cutting board on top of a pulled out drawer or by arranging a wooden cutting board on your lap. If your writing surface is too high, use a lapboard.
- Make a low movable work station from a two-shelf utility cart. The lower shelf folds up and leaves leg room so you can sit to work on the top shelf.
- Find a hospital overbed table in a thrift shop. You can adjust the height to accommodate sitting or standing positions.
- For gardening, have a handyman create planter beds which allow you to sit comfortably while you work on your flowers and vegetables.

Correct Seating is Critical

A properly fitted chair supports your back and thighs, aids circulation in your legs, and reduces fatigue and back pain. The seat height and backrest should both be adjustable. The seat depth should allow your back to be snug against the backrest, with your feet supported on the floor. If raising the chair high enough to have a low work surface causes your feet to dangle, use a large 3-ring binder notebook to support your feet. Hips and knees should not be flexed more than ninety degrees to allow adequate circulation in the legs. Sit on a wedge seat cushion with the high edge in back.

To prevent computer fatigue, put the keyboard just below elbow level and the monitor high enough so your head stays erect. For most individuals, the top of the screen should be at eye level, but if you wear bifocals or trifocals, the screen needs to be lower. Use a copy holder attached to the side of your monitor to hold your copy at eye level. Place a wrist platform in front of the keyboard to support your wrists in a neutral position. This prevents carpal tunnel syndrome as well as muscle fatigue.

Organizing Your Kitchen

Meal preparation and cleanup take a lot of time and energy and have to be done more often than any other chore. So let's begin with making the kitchen user-friendly. A little arranging can make the difference.

The principle is to "rack 'em and stack 'em." Store everyday dishes in stacks of their own kind. Don't put small saucers on top of big ones, or small bowls inside of larger bowls. Purchase vinyl-coated wire racks for stacking same-size plates, saucers, bowls, etc. Stack pots and skillets one layer deep, so you don't have to lift the top items to get at the bottom one. Wire racks are available for either horizontal or vertical storage of individual skillets or pans.

Use one-motion storage of grocery items. If your pantry shelves are deep enough to hold more than one layer, make the second (and third) layer the same as the first. That means you put a can of peaches behind another can of peaches, not behind a can of tomatoes. This way you can see all your supplies at a glance without having to remove the front items.

Utilize stacking storage bins on wheels and adjustable shelf units that hook over pantry doors. Store condiments on lazy susans. Put infrequently-used items on lazy susans and employ a reacher for turning and retrieving items from upper shelves. One and two level sliding racks, bins, baskets and shelf trays make base cabinets usable for dishes, utensils, food staples, and cleaning supplies.

Keep supplies close to the area of first use. For instance, saucepans are usually used first at the sink because you put water in them before taking them to the stove.

An angled mirror against the wall over the stove allows you to see what's cooking on the back burners while you're seated.

The Bathroom

The bathroom is the most-used room in the home and the easiest to make user-friendly. Raised toilet seats can be purchased in many different styles and are easy to secure to existing toilets. A safety frame which attaches at the back of the toilet seat has handles for pushing up, if additional assistance is needed. You can also use an over-the-toilet commode with safety rails and adjustable legs. Caution: Towel bars are not designed for pulling up one's body weight. Use grab bars instead.

Tub baths require muscle power that some of us don't possess. With minimal leg weakness, you might need only a little assist from a safety rail which mounts easily on the outside of the tub or a grab bar attached to the wall. If getting up is really difficult, switch to showering and sit on a bath bench and utilize a flexible shower hose.

Replace sliding bathtub doors with a shower curtain. The doors, tracks, and tub are difficult to clean. If you need to transfer from a wheelchair, the doors don't allow space to swing your legs over. Install safety treads to prevent slips in the tub or shower stall.

Grab bars are essential safety features for tubs and showers. Soap dishes, like towel racks, are not designed for pulling oneself up. Nowadays there is a selection of attractive, decorative grab bars that actually improve the bathroom decor while providing the needed support.

Round faucet handles which require force to turn can cause stress to small finger joints. Replace them with long-lever handles which can be pushed with your palm or forearm.

Throughout the House

Avoid deep-pile carpets with thick padding. Wheelchair users find deep pile difficult for maneuvering, and ambulators with mobility problems can have difficulty keeping their balance as they sink with each step. Avoid using throw rugs. They can slip or catch as you move. Ceramic tile floors are slippery when wet; vinyl, wood or cork are better options.

Place electric outlets at least 18 inches above the floor. Install light switches near the entryway to each room so you don't have to walk or wheel in the dark.

Install telephone extensions in as many rooms as possible. Request a portable telephone from your local phone company, which provides a whole range of adaptive telephone aids to individuals with disabilities. They will even send a representative to your home to analyze your situation and supply you with free equipment.

Plan ahead to minimize trips. Install floor-to-ceiling pole shelves over the toilet tank in each bathroom for stacking towels and washcloths. Store sheets and pillowcases in each bedroom where they are used. Use your central linen closet just for storing items you need occasionally. Hook up your washer and dryer near the bedrooms and bathrooms if possible. Most of the laundry is generated in these areas.

Duplicate supplies or small equipment which is used in different areas. For instance, store cleanser and sponges under each sink in the house; keep a broom and dustpan in several locations.

Eliminate stairs. If you are ambulatory but have lower extremity weakness, you must eliminate stairs from your daily activities. This is probably the single most important adaptation you can make. When you walk, your entire body weight is borne on the sole of your foot, a very small area. This means that you are putting three times your body weight on your foot during the weight-bearing phase of walking. Going up steps is much more stressful than that. Some years ago, efficiency experts determined how much energy (in the form of calories) was used by healthy individuals in performing various activities. Their results showed that compared to lying still:

- Sitting at rest took 30 percent more energy
- Walking 2.6 miles per hour took 160 percent more energy
- Walking 3.75 miles per hour took 290 percent more energy
- Walking downstairs took 372 percent more energy
- Walking upstairs took 1336 percent more energy.

Stair climbing uses over eight times more energy than moderate walking. If going up stairs is so energy-consuming for healthy individuals, you can see why it is essential for people with a chronic condition to eliminate this activity.

Even a few exterior steps, or one steep step, can make you feel like a prisoner in your own home. Ramps facilitate independence for the ambulatory as well as the wheelchair-user. Properly graded ramps, which are one foot long for each one inch of rise, permit comfortable wheelchair propelling and allow ambulators to pull loads up and down on a luggage or grocery cart.

If at all possible, move out of a multi-level dwelling. If this is not possible, try to relocate most of your daily activities to one level. A stair elevator, although expensive, may be tax deductible if prescribed by a physician.

Store items that are used together in one place. Collecting supplies from different locations wastes time and energy. Plan activities so as to eliminate extra trips between table and counter, room to room, or up and down stairs.

Your Automobile

This is the biggest and most challenging piece of equipment you use. A vehicle with an automatic transmission and with power steering, locks, and windows is indispensable. Opening the door, getting in and out, switching the ignition key, maintaining a grip on the steering wheel, keeping your body and arms in a good position are just some of the problems presented to individuals with weak extremities.

Getting up and down from low-slung bucket seats is a chore when your legs are weak. Ideally the seat should be at hip height to facilitate sliding in and out. Small pickup trucks and most minivans have seats at this height. Full-size vans are too high and require a step up to get inside. Unless you need a full-size van for transporting an electric wheelchair, think carefully before purchasing this model.

If you have a choice of seat covering, vinyl is easier to slide on than cloth. Continuously gripping the steering wheel can cause pain and fatigue in the hand and elbow muscles. Purchase steering wheel covers with padding and lacing to enlarge the wheel and provide traction. Although lambswool covers look good, they can become slippery and may force you to grip harder to steer safely.

You can prevent shoulder fatigue with armrests to support your elbows. They are easy to fabricate with high-density foam you can purchase from an upholstery shop.

SIMPLIFY YOUR WORK

Don't put away the most frequently used pans or skillets. After each use, wash and let them dry on top of the stove. Let dishes drip dry in a rack instead of towel-drying and then set the table for the next meal. When boiling pasta or vegetables, put the food into a round stainless steel mesh basket with a handle (available from mail order houses) which can be easily lifted out of the boiling water. After the water cools, slide the pot to the sink and empty it.

Use the principle of gravity. It is easier to let things fall down instead of putting them down. Place your cutting board on the counter next to the sink and set a bowl in the sink. The chopped food can then be pushed off the board into the bowl instead of being put in by handfuls. For wheelchair or electric cart users, a bowl in your lap allows you to push the food into it right from the cutting board.

Prepare double recipes for items such as meat loaves, muffins, etc., and store half for use at another time. There are a wide variety of convenience foods available today including: prepared salads and vegetables from your supermarket salad bar; frozen chopped onions; canned soups for sauces, TV dinners (some are delicious and healthy); and "carry-out." Do chores the same way each time. Repetition increases efficiency.

How about entertaining? Your social life is important, and it doesn't need to wear you out. Have a potluck. Or order a party tray from the supermarket—there are lots of choices, from cold cuts and sandwiches to fruit and vegetable platters. At holiday time, some supermarkets offer a cooked turkey or ham dinner with all the trimmings. Use paper plates, cups, napkins and tablecloths. Place a large plastic trash bag where your guests can empty their own garbage. When everyone is through eating, close the bag with a wire twisty and ask a nondisabled guest to carry it outside.

It is important to eliminate extra trips. When grocery shopping, mentally divide the cart into four areas. In one section put frozen or need-to-be-frozen foods. In another section put items that need refrigeration. Place canned goods and staples in the third section. Put cleaning supplies, paper products and personal care items in the fourth section. Ask the checker to pack lightly and to place each category into separate bags. When you get home and load the bags into your collapsible cart, you only need to make one trip each to the refrigerator, freezer and cupboard. If you are really fatigued, just put away the freezer and refrigerator foods and take a rest before you finish the job.

Use Energy-Efficient Equipment

Energy efficient equipment can be found in most houseware departments. A microwave oven can decrease the number of dishes used for cooking, serving and storing. Take advantage of dishes that can be used for all these steps. An electric knife carves many things besides turkeys and roasts. It also slices hard cheese, vegetables, fruits, etc. A jar chopper cuts with pressure from the palm; no need to grip a knife with your fingers. To reduce mechanical stress on the finger joints, use an electric can opener. A cordless can opener is lightweight, rechargeable, and requires no pressure to operate once the cutter has been activated. A piece of non-skid material under the can keeps it from drifting. Other uses for non-skid material are holding bowls in place while you mix food or as a place mat to keep your plate from sliding when cutting food.

There are many knives available now which are ergonomically correct—that is, the handle is enlarged and angled to keep the wrist in neutral position while cutting food. They are ideal for persons with arthritis, tendinitis or hand weakness. Originally from Sweden, they are available now in many home stores. Some other readily available items which make life easier are gardening pruners that have a ratchet mechanism, electric scissors, and electric staplers.

Use a salad shooter or mini food processor to prepare vegetables. Large food processors require too much cleanup. Don't use heavy dishes or cookware. Switch to Corelle and lightweight, non-stick skillets.

Now some housework tips (if you must do your own cleaning). Pushing an upright vacuum cleaner is much easier than pulling a canister type and provides something to lean against. Some models are lightweight and have the attachments placed at waist level. Eliminate bending when you sweep or mop by using a long-handled dustpan and a mop that doesn't need hand wringing.

Adaptive Equipment

Adaptive equipment is usually ordered from special vendors, as opposed to the energy-efficient equipment which is available in many stores. You will find a list of adaptive equipment vendors in the Appendix. However, some mail order catalogs and pharmacies now offer some types of adaptive equipment.

Reachers are one of the great all-purpose pieces of equipment. Besides picking items off the floor and down from shelves, they can help you with other household chores and assist with lower extremity dressing. They come in two different grip styles: scissor grip and squeeze grip. Do not purchase scissor grip reachers for any reason. They are awkward, uncomfortable, require strong finger and wrist muscles, have poor leverage, and require the use of two hands for maintaining grip on large or heavy objects.

Reachers with a squeeze grip come in enough models to suit almost any person's requirements. Some have rubber claws for securely gripping slippery objects and magnetic tips for lifting small metallic objects. Some have changeable claw angles or locking claws. All can be used with one hand. One new style has a wrist support for weaker grasps, and another model requires no finger control but uses a small amount of wrist extension to close the claws. There is a reacher for every purpose. Choose one that matches your strength and ability, the distances you need to reach, and the type of objects you need to hold. You may need different types of reachers in several locations.

The following aids can help to compensate for weak grasp or pinch, or for accomplishing tasks with only one hand:

- The buttonhook-zipper pull combination helps to manipulate small fastenings. If your grip is extremely weak, a quad-quip buttoner-zipper combination fits over the hand and eliminates gripping.
- A utensil holder fits around the palm and has a pouch to eliminate the need to grip brushes, writing implements, feeding utensils, etc. A rocker knife cuts food with one hand by rocking the sharp curved bottom blade back and forth.
- Food preparation with one hand is made easier with a cutting board with two stainless steel nails to hold the food securely, a roller knife (similar to a pizza cutter), a one-handed egg beater, and a self-contained grater with suction feet which has a bin to catch the food. Other kitchen devices are one-handed jar openers, suction bottle brushes, and pan holders.

- Door knob extensions provide extra leverage for easier opening and install easily without removing the door knob. Also available is a portable door knob turner for when you leave home. Car door openers will open either push-button or lift-type door handles and key holders give extra leverage in turning locks.
- You can easily build up handles on combs, toothbrushes, pens, etc., by slipping a foam hair curler over the handle. Cylindrical hard foam handles are also available for various utensils. You can purchase cylindrical foam by the yard with a choice of outside diameters and inner bores.
- If you have difficulty reaching your feet, there are many aids to facilitate dressing: dressing sticks, sock aids, long-handled shoe horns, and elastic shoelaces that turn a laced shoe into a slip-on shoe.

Community Resources

Some supermarkets have electric scooters for disabled customers to use while shopping. If your local store doesn't offer this service, let the manager know that accommodating the disabled customers in his area will increase his profits.

Vote by absentee ballot. If your ballot doesn't include a request for an absentee ballot, call your local Registrar of Voters to request permanent Absentee Ballot status. You will automatically be sent an absentee ballot before each election.

Order postage stamps by mail or telephone. For the former, complete a postage-free order form, enclose a check and leave it for your mail carrier. Orders are usually returned within three business days, and there are no extra charges. Stamps by Phone takes Visa or Mastercard orders 24 hours a day at 1-800-782-6724 and charges a modest fee to cover credit card and phone charges.

CONCLUSIONS

In conclusion, energy conservation is a lifelong process. These suggestions are to help you analyze your daily behavior so you can select the modifications that are appropriate to your particular lifestyle.

You may decide to eliminate some of the activities that no longer seem essential and modify some of those that are valuable to you. There is good news, however. Studies have shown that polio survivors who have implemented energy conservation strategies did not lose further muscle strength and, in fact, reported improvement in pain and fatigue. You can take an active part in your own physical well-being. After all, the purpose in conserving your energy is to enable you to continue doing whatever is most meaningful, most fun and most satisfying.

6

Lifestyle Changes: Taking Charge

LAURA K. SMITH

Just as there was no cure for acute poliomyelitis, there is no cure for post-polio syndrome (PPS). Nevertheless, people with acute poliomyelitis were treated to prevent, alleviate, or correct the problems or symptoms they had. So too the people with PPS can be treated to prevent and alleviate their new problems of fatigue, pain, or weakness. Most of the symptoms and their causes in each stage of poliomyelitis (acute, convalescent, period of stability, and now PPS) are different. Therefore, the treatments can be expected to be different. Treatment used in the acute stage was not appropriate in the convalescent stage, and that used in the convalescent or chronic phase is not appropriate for the symptoms of PPS. For example, the major treatment for increasing muscle strength during the convalescent stage was muscle reeducation. These exercises were carried out for each weak or paralyzed muscle in the body. The physical therapist moved the extremity three times in the direction that the muscle would pull when it contracted, passing his or her finger on the skin over the muscle. The patient would then try to contract the muscle in three trials. A great deal of attention was paid to the avoidance of substitution made by stronger muscles. Substitution permitted the strong muscles to get stronger; the weak muscles would not be activated to regain strength. Muscle reeducation occupied a great deal of treatment time, but three isolated contractions of individual muscles did not constitute a strenuous workout.

After approximately six months to nine months from onset of poliomyelitis, the muscle test scores gradually improved and then leveled off. It was thought that the damaged motor neurons had made maximum recovery. The treatment then changed to resistive exercise for building muscle strength together with intensive work on functional activities such as transfers, walking, or climbing stairs. If at any time there was a decrease in muscle strength or the muscle failed to increase as expected, it was thought that the program was too strenuous and the program was decreased.

The period of functional stability of poliomyelitis began from one year to two years after onset of the disease. In this phase, many polio survivors were able to develop incredible strength in some parts of their bodies. Women have reported being competitive with men in arm-wrestling. The incredible strength and functional ability resulted from the combination of axon sprouting and muscle fiber enlargement or hypertrophy described in Chapter One. This condition could occur in muscles that had *subclinical* or undetected polio and in muscles with mild to moderate weakness at onset. Hypertrophy could not occur in paralyzed muscles. These strength gains were accomplished by long term: (1) heavy resistive exercise (weight lifting); (2) competitive sports such as tennis, basketball, or track; (3) heavy manual labor; (4) propelling a manual wheelchair and making body transfers with the arms; or (5) walking with crutches and braces.

When the new problems of PPS began to occur, many people turned again to strenuous exercise workouts only to be puzzled to find that their symptoms did not improve. More often, the pain, fatigue, or new weakness became worse. The cause of these problems is different from the cause of pain and weakness in the earlier stages of polio; therefore, the treatment is different. Management of PPS places emphasis on taking the load off the muscles by using energy conservation techniques, lifestyle modifications, and building a reserve capacity.

The most successful treatment program for PPS is survivor and family education, which teaches the survivors the principles of, and methods for, self-management of their bodies. The purpose of this chapter is to give survivors information and resources that can help them to develop self-directed management programs for PPS.

MANAGEMENT OF LIFESTYLE CHANGES IN PPS

An important part of the treatment of PPS is education of the survivors and their families in a self-management treatment program.

In the early phases of polio there was little, if any, patient or parental education except for exercise programs. In contrast, a great deal of information is now available about acute polio, the effects on the body, and the relationship to PPS. Information needs to be provided about the effects of the poliovirus on the nerve cells and muscles, the widespread invasion of the virus in the brain and spinal cord, the possible existence of polio involvement in extremities thought to be unaffected, the processes of muscle strength recovery in the convalescent stage, the effects of years of compensatory movements on the body, and prominent theories on the causes of PPS. (See Chapter One for details.)

Become an Intelligent Consumer

The first step is to learn about PPS and the resources available for help. Many are listed in Appendix A of this book. The PPS support groups are particularly rich sources of information. One of the main reasons for the need to have an understanding of PPS is that few health professionals have knowledge of the effects of polio or PPS. Acute polio disappeared in this country in the early 1960s because of the protection given by the Salk and Sabin vaccines. The subject of poliomyelitis was reduced in medical classes and textbooks to a mere passing mention. Thus, it has been difficult for polio survivors to get appropriate medical care. Today, the survivors need to provide the interested health professional with references and resources for information. Such need develops, for example, with dental surgery when local or general anesthesia is to be used. It is wise to give these busy practitioners a copy of a pertinent medical article or even a copy of this book. If the health professional shows interest, other articles can be provided. Also, family members, employers, or friends require orientation to the condition and, in particular, to the modifications that would be helpful.

Obtain a Comprehensive Medical Evaluation

The diagnosis of PPS is difficult and challenging. The diagnostic procedure is reviewed in Chapter Two. It is important to have a complete medical evaluation because the symptoms of PPS are similar to other conditions, or they may be combined with the symptoms of other conditions. Self-diagnosis is dangerous. The best source for survivor and family education is the comprehensive medical evaluation available at more than 60 post-polio clinics found throughout the United States. In these clinics, the individual will receive a comprehensive evaluation by health professionals specializing in PPS.

Many people who are interested in finding out if they have PPS, or are at risk of the condition, are unable to go to a post-polio clinic because of distance, time, medical plan, personal preference, or expense. Many physicians are interested in treating people with PPS, but they are hard to find. During the polio epidemics, orthopedists and pediatricians were the primary care physicians for those with polio. Today, the most knowledgeable physician group on PPS is that specializing in physical medicine and rehabilitation (physiatrists). Many support groups keep a list of names of physicians who are recommended by their members. If a survivor has a physician who is not interested in PPS or in learning about it and that person's problems, the best advice is to seek out someone who is interested and can be helpful.

Depending on the facility or the physician, treatment recommendations may vary from a simple admonition such as, "Don't do too much," to a detailed list of 20 or more specific interventions. In the former type of recommendation, the survivor must figure out what to do. The latter type usually advises how to carry out each recommendation, but their combined enormity overwhelms the survivor. The best advice for the individual is to pick one intervention that seems easy to do, incorporate it into his or her lifestyle, and then pick another that appears possible, and proceed from that point. For example, weight reduction is a common suggestion that is extremely helpful when it can be carried out. Weight control, however, is one of the most difficult recommendations to achieve. It is not wise to start with the most difficult. Instead, lower the priority of weight reduction on the list. As benefits are gained from the other recommendations, it becomes easier to take on the more difficult ones.

Preserve and Protect Limited Muscle and Joint Capacities

PPS symptoms of abnormal body fatigue, muscle and joint pain, and new muscle weakness are considered to be partly caused by long-term overuse of muscles and joints at high levels of their capacity. In this way, post-polio survivors have been able to compete successfully with people who have full nerve-muscle complements. For example, in walking, any type of limp requires more energy than normal walking for the same speed; walking with crutches and braces may require two times to four times the energy of normal walking. The limp may also cause overstretching of ligaments and joint wear and tear. In addition, polio survivors may contract some of their muscles continuously in walking. During normal walking, the muscles contract and relax during each step somewhat like the heart when it pumps blood. It is only during the relaxation phase, when the pressure is off the small blood vessels, that the essential exchange of nutrients and waste products of the muscle can occur. Continuous contraction leads to inadequate nourishment of the muscle and decreased endurance.

After 20 years to 30 years or more, the muscles and joints cannot continue to operate at these high levels of their already limited capacity. Forcing their continued operation leads to further pain and inability to perform functional activities. As a result, the survivor decreases his or her activity and participation in work, family, and social functions. Most survivors opt to make changes by learning to maintain their function by doing things the easy way, including taking advantage of modern comforts and technology and alternate methods of locomotion.

The following two subsections focus on two activities polio survivors need to accomplish to ensure the preservation and protection of muscles and joints.

Inventory Activities

Make a detailed list of all activities at home and work and in the community. Start when arising in the morning and continue throughout the day. Indicate the amount of time, distance, and/or number of times for a typical day. Survivors who walk should purchase a pedometer and measure how many miles they walk per day or week. One lady, who stated she did not do anything any more, found she walked three miles per day inside her home! Those pushing a manual wheelchair should also measure distance and specifically list the number of ramps and slopes ascended and the number of transfers performed. Remember to include in a separate area periodic activities, such as big family dinners, caring for grandchildren, trips, and vacations. Often such events can be so exhausting and physically stressful, they become a horror for the polio survivor.

Another technique that can be helpful is to analyze and assign a priority to each of the activities and address the following questions:

- Can the number of trips be decreased without reducing the function?
- Can a less strenuous way be used to perform the activity?
- What modern comforts and technology, including electronics and motorization, can reduce the energy expenditure of the activity?
- Can the activity be separated into parts to be done several times in a day or week with rest periods or a different activity between?
- What other people can perform some or all of this activity? For example, does the survivor need to push the lawnmower and hold the weed eater? Is there a family member, a young neighborhood entrepreneur, or a yardman who could do as well with a little supervision? Or, if the lawn is large enough, the survivor might enjoy the luxury of a riding mower.

This inventory and evaluation of activities together with other recommendations should form a map for energy conservation.

Weight Control

Together with the program of energy conservation, it is important to recognize that as activity declines, the amount of food intake should decrease as well. Weight gain will follow if the amount of food is not decreased. Increased weight in turn increases the load on the muscles and joints, leading to further fatigue, pain, and muscle weakness. Attention needs to focus on eating low-fat foods and decreasing the size of servings. It is important not to skip a meal such as breakfast. This strategy causes the body to think it is starving. The body then slows the metabolism and stores food, which leads to further weight gain.

Exercise for the purpose of weight reduction is not usually an option for those with PPS because they are already suffering from overuse of their muscles and cannot tolerate the strenuous exercises needed to lose weight. Thus, weight control may need to be accomplished by diet alone. Daily or at least weekly weight checks are important, if possible. If weight control cannot be managed, the survivor needs to get the help of a dietician. Remember, however, that this person may need educational materials about PPS and the reasons the survivor cannot add additional exercise. The polio survivor needs to make permanent modifications of lifelong nutritional habits without resorting to exercise. Although difficult to achieve, weight loss is probably the single, most effective method for taking the load off the muscles. Many survivors do so successfully.

Treatment of Fatigue, Muscle Pain, and New Muscle Weakness

While energy conservation techniques, nonfatiguing functional activities, and weight control are the primary recommendations for the treatment of fatigue, muscle pain, and new muscle weakness, specific treatment interventions also exist for each of these symptoms.

PPS generalized fatigue is an abnormal and unique type of fatigue. It can vary from an occasional episode to a daily afternoon *slump*, to being tired all the time. The fatigue can be so bad that the survivor goes into a cycle of waking up fatigued, going to work, coming home to go to bed, and spending weekends in bed.

Learn techniques of relaxation or imagery to maximize rest periods. In addition to energy conservation techniques, rest periods are important for relief of PPS fatigue. Recommendations often include one hour of rest or sleep per day at home or at work. For more severe fatigue, rest periods need to be more frequent. Many say, however, that they spend all the time they are supposed to be resting thinking about what they are not doing. To make these rest periods more effective, the survivor needs to learn the art of relaxation. Audio tapes for relaxation and meditation or massage music are helpful mediums for achieving a deeper, more effective relaxed state. These tapes can be purchased at health food stores and upscale book stores. It is best to have an automatic reverse cassette to avoid abrupt interruption of relaxation; earphones are important in consideration of other people.

If energy conservation techniques and rest periods do not decrease fatigue and muscle pain, the working person should consider taking two months to three months of temporary medical leave. This type of leave provides the opportunity to see the effect of a more intensive modification of activities and doing things the easy way. Homemakers are considered to be working persons; arrangements need to be made for them to take medical leave.

The muscle pain reported by survivors with PPS is deep, aching and diffuse. This pain appears in muscles weakened earlier in the acute episode of polio. When the pain appears in extremities the survivor considers to be strong or not to have been affected by polio, it is frightening. Even people who were diagnosed as having non-paralytic polio in the acute phase have this type of muscle pain. This finding is not surprising because slight muscle weaknesses were not discovered due to the emergency epidemic conditions, the need for hospital beds, and the lack of trained physical therapists to perform detailed and accurate manual muscle tests. Chapter Two describes the phenomenon of persons who believed they had no polio in certain muscles, but now have positive symptoms in those limbs or signs of old polio revealed by electromyographic examinations.

PPS survivors say that their deep aching muscle pain does not respond to the usual pain medications, but that warm water provides a temporary relief. Many, however, brag about taking a bath in water as hot as they can stand it. Such high temperatures may cause injury to the body and have little effect in producing long-term decrease in this type of muscle pain. The high temperature creates a burning pain that blocks the lesser muscle pain temporarily. Such hot baths cause an increase in the body temperature and heart rate and produce a debilitating exhaustion. If the person is going to be submerged, such as sitting in a hot tub or spa with water up to the neck, the water temperature should be warm (96°F to 98°F) and exposure limited to 20 minutes. If only a leg or arm is submerged, the water temperature may be up to 105°F.

Avoid unessential physical activity. The best way to relieve muscle pain is to take the load off the muscles. Examples for the lower extremities include avoiding stairs, low chairs and deep knee bends and using elevators, elevated chairs, reserved parking, shower stools and weight control principles. Decreasing the load on the upper extremities requires not only limitations on lifting, pushing, and pulling but also attention to low-level repetitive activities, such as using the computer; sewing and handwork; holding a book or magazine for reading; and gesturing with the hands when talking. Decreasing workloads on muscles sufficiently to eliminate muscle pain may require using an orthosis (brace), and/or limiting walking to the home or workplace, and using a motorized cart for distance locomotion.

Recovery from the PPS type of muscle pain and fatigue can take from months to a year. The amount of time depends on the severity of the pain and fatigue, the length of time these problems have been present, and the survivor's ability to incorporate major lifestyle changes. One polio clinic found that pain and fatigue were decreased or absent in all of those who were able to incorporate recommendations into their lifestyle. Of those who could not make the lifestyle changes, the pain was the same or worse in 85 percent and the fatigue was the same or worse in 100 percent.

Types of New Muscle Weakness

Three types of new muscle weakness occur in polio survivors: (1) normal decline of muscle strength with aging, (2) weakness from long-term overuse of muscles beyond their capacity, and (3) muscle weakness from disuse.

Decline of Muscle Strength with Aging

It is well known that athletes have a decline in maximum strength and skill as they get older. They become less competitive in their sport; but this loss of strength does not cause any loss of ability to perform daily activities, most of which only require 10 percent to 20 percent of maximum capacity. The same type of loss of strength happens to people who are not athletes. Measurement of maximum grip strength in over 1000 active people showed the highest average grip strength occurred at 35 years of age (130 pounds for men and 80 pounds for women). At age 65, the average grip strength decreased by 25 percent to 100 pounds for men and 60 pounds for women. This type of muscle strength decline also occurs with people who had polio.

People who had paralytic polio are very much like superathletes in that they operate at high levels of their muscle capacity to carry out daily activities and work. The polio "athletes," however, have a markedly decreased maximum muscle capacity. When they lose even a small amount of muscle strength with age, it may become very noticeable. As a result, they lose a proportional ability to perform activities of daily living such as walking, writing, or breathing. This decline in ability may be reported by the survivor as muscle fatigue, loss of endurance, or new muscle weakness.

Overuse Weakness and Overload Exercise

The second type of muscle weakness in persons with PPS results from an overuse of muscles relative to their capacity. New weakness occurs in muscles that are active but have polio and in strong extremities that were not thought to have had polio. For example, one survivor stated, "My polio leg is fine, but my good right leg is getting weaker and painful." When he stood, all the weight was supported by his right leg. On the other hand, people with use of all of their muscles have many standing postures, first on one leg, then on the other, and then on both legs. This man, however, has only *one* standing posture. In addition to overloading the right leg in standing, this limb was doing double duty with every step in walking, going up and down stairs, sitting down and rising, or getting up from the floor. To decrease pain and fatigue in the good leg, a knee-ankle-foot-orthosis (KAFO or a long leg brace) was recommended for the *left leg*. This brace permitted him to bear weight on the left leg and brace when he stood and to relax the right leg. By using the KAFO he also reduced the continuous work of the right leg in walking and in going up and down stairs. After several weeks, his low back pain was eliminated because he was now walking in a more erect position. Recommendations for lifestyle modifications for this man included using reserved parking, limiting distance walking, avoiding stairs, elevating chairs and commode seats in the home, and avoiding getting down on the floor except in an emergency. With all these lifestyle changes, the weakness and pain in his strong right leg were relieved and he was able to continue working. Ongoing issues, such as weight control and decreasing the energy requirements of gardening and going to sports events, became easier to attack. With such a program, the rate of decline in muscle strength can be slowed.

A common concern of polio survivors is the effect exercise has on these muscles working at high levels of their capacity and getting weaker. If normal muscles are caused to exercise or work in an overload situation (to maximum ability and then more) for a period of weeks and months, the muscles respond with an increase in performance and size. During the early convalescent stage of polio, the overload principle was not recommended until the person was one year from onset. It is believed that such strenuous work stopped the muscle recovery that was occurring. However, once the first year was passed, strenuous workouts were acceptable and used extensively. Many survivors achieved incredible strength through the dual processes of sprouting and hypertrophy of muscle fibers (Chapter One).

Thirty years to fifty years later, when the muscles seemed to be getting weak, painful, and fatigued, the survivors turned again to the overload principle. They started working out, joined aerobic classes, began swimming laps, increased their workouts, and started using the stairs at work. Although the symptoms were getting worse, it was difficult for the survivors to think that the worsening of the symptoms might be related to the additional exercise or work. Overworked and already fatigued muscles cannot respond to the overload principle with increased performance and hypertrophy; rather, these muscles respond with decreased performance and pain. In some instances, a muscle or part of a muscle may become visibly smaller (post-polio muscular atrophy).

Preserve muscle capacity for important function, work, family, and social activities. It is best to stop exercises designed to increase muscle strength as a part of lifestyle changes to unload the muscles. After the fatigue and muscle pain are gone and a reserve capacity has been built up, carefully monitored aerobic and strengthening exercises can be evaluated for their benefit to present and future activity. Very mild exercises may be helpful when there is still muscle pain and fatigue. Easy underwater exercises (nonresistive) in a warm pool, relaxation or meditation exercises, and body awareness techniques, such as Feldenkrais exercises, may all be helpful.

Muscle Weakness from Disuse

Muscle weakness from disuse occurs when muscles have not been used or have been underused. This weakness can happen with cast immobilization of an arm or leg to heal a fracture or after bedrest for the flu, surgery, or illness. In addition to muscle weakness in the extremities, bedrest causes deconditioning of the muscles of the heart, lungs, and blood vessels (cardiovascular and respiratory systems). People with PPS decondition more rapidly and recover more slowly from bedrest and immobilization than people with full complements of spinal motor neurons. When a survivor has one of these debilitating conditions, it is a good idea to have a reconditioning exercise program started as soon as possible. Even a partial conditioning program while still at bedrest can be helpful.

A reconditioning program consists of exercises and functional activities, such as sitting up, standing, or walking. Activities are designed to maintain the present level of muscle activity and, in a carefully graduated manner, to challenge and increase muscle strength and aerobic fitness back to the pre-illness or pre-injury level. These programs are usually provided by physical and/or occupational therapists. Most physical and occupational therapists, however, are unfamiliar with polio. Here is another situation when it is crucial to provide health professionals with information on polio and PPS. It is most important to show or describe the ways that the survivor performs daily activities such as transfers, rising up from chairs, or walking. This transfer information is necessary because each polio survivor has a unique pattern of muscle weakness and joint range of motion, and each has developed special ways that are best suited to his or her ability to perform functional activities.

If disuse weakness is suspected, a rule of thumb for the therapist in estimating the intensity and amount of exercise or activity appropriate for the survivor is: (1) estimate the intensity (load) that the survivor can tolerate and then apply one-half the load, (2) reduce the estimated number of repetitions by one-half, and (3) double the time of the estimated rest periods. If fatigue resolves in less than 30 minutes, does not recur in the next two days, and muscle pain does not increase, the program can be gradually increased. The appearance of muscle pain or fatigue indicates an overload and requires reevaluation of the exercises and other activities in which the survivor may have engaged.

Similar problems of fatigue and weakness can occur in the muscles of respiration, swallowing, or speech. The survivors who had bulbar polio need to be aware of the possibility of new weakness in the muscles of respiration or swallowing. Any type of history of breathing or swallowing problems in the acute phase, such as, "They kept the iron lung outside my room, but I did not need it," indicates the possibility of polio involvement of the muscles of respiration or swallowing. These topics are discussed in more detail in Chapter Two.

MANAGEMENT OF MUSCLE AND JOINT INJURIES

Post-polio survivors, whether they have PPS or not, are subject to neuro-musculo-skeletal injuries (nerve-muscle-bone) that cause sufficient pain to interfere with function. This type of pain is more localized than the deep and diffuse muscle pain of PPS. Another difference is that PPS muscle pain tends to be continuous, while the musculoskeletal injury pain usually can be decreased or increased with different positions, muscle contractions, motions, or pressures. Some of these injuries can be the result of falls and trauma, but most of the problems are caused by long-term, repetitive, abnormal forces on body structures. Abnormal forces occur because of muscle weakness or paralysis and the amazing ability of the body to try to substitute other muscles or ligaments to compensate for muscle losses. The problem is that the substitution is not exactly the same as the forces produced by normal muscles and joints. Substitute muscles may have to pull at an angle and apply a greater force in a different direction. In mechanical terms, this situation would be like running an automobile on three cylinders (instead of six) with the front end out of alignment. In the body, these abnormal forces occur during postures such as sitting, standing, or sleeping and activities such as walking, standing up from a chair, or typewriting. In time, however, these abnormal forces cause uneven wear and tear on joint structures (osteoarthritis), overstretching and weakening of ligaments and muscles, tightening of fascia (sheaths of fibrous tissue surrounding muscles and joints), and pinching of tissues (including nerves). In many cases, if these conditions are untreated, further loss of functional ability will result.

Unfortunately, many post-polio survivors and health professionals look upon these pain problems as just arthritis, a condition one has to learn to live with. The pain is treated with medication and heat. This treatment, however, provides temporary relief. The condition becomes worse and more difficult to correct, and another impairment is added that the survivor has to compensate for.

Repetitive Stress Injuries in Post-Polio Survivors

Most of the pain problems experienced by polio survivors are like the repetitive stress injuries (RSI) or cumulative trauma of the workplace or sports. Carpal tunnel syndrome (CTS) is associated with long-term computer use by nonpolio persons. In people with PPS, there is a very high frequency of CTS in those using round handgrips on crutches or canes. These assistive devices produce point pressure on weight-bearing surfaces of the hands and compression of a nerve at the wrist. Untreated CTS can cause loss of sensation and muscle strength in the hand. Tennis elbow is named after injuries associated with the backhand stroke in tennis. The pain is on the outside of the elbow. The injury, however, is caused by overuse of the muscles that open the fingers or lift the wrist. Activity causing this kind of injury is low-level repetitive motion from hammering to handwork such as needlepoint. Other RSI injuries to the upper extremity in people with PPS include gamekeeper's thumb (loosening of ligaments at the base of the thumb causing pain and inability to grasp or pinch objects) and Little League elbow (muscle pain on the inner side of the elbow). These two RSIs can be caused by long-term propulsion of a manual wheelchair.

The shoulder takes a beating from long-term use of a manual wheelchair or walking with crutches and braces. Two of the most common shoulder RSIs are: (1) bicipital tendonitis, a fraying and pain of the long tendon of the biceps muscle (in the arm), as the tendon crosses the shoulder bone; and (2) rotator cuff injuries to the muscles that attach around the joint capsule of the shoulder. In addition, there is a high frequency of abnormal head and neck postures with referral of pain to the head, shoulder, arm, or hand.

In the trunk and lower extremities, one of the most common RSIs in polio survivors is sacroileitis (sacroiliac joint or SIJ inflammation and SIJ pain). Two SI joints join the trunk to the pelvis. These two joints are formed by the upside-down triangular sacral bone, wedged on each side between the two iliac or pelvic bones. The top of the sacrum forms the base for the spine. The tailbone is attached to the lower part of the sacrum (apex of the triangle). Motion in the SIJs is small, about ¼-inch in young adults. In women during pregnancy, the ligaments of the joints relax and permit greater motion of the SIJs. These ligaments do not always tighten up properly after the birth, resulting in excessive motion.

Injury to the SI joints in persons with PPS is most frequently related to walking and caused by long-term uneven and excessive forces on the joints. Such abnormal forces occur with hip muscle weakness, a short leg, or pain in the leg or foot. These problems cause excessive sideward movement of the trunk on the weight-bearing leg during walking. This excessive motion causes repetitive abnormal forces on the SI joints with each step.

Other common RSIs of post-polio survivors are trochanteric bursitis (inflammation of the bone on the side of the hip), which causes pain when lying on the side or walking; and, patello-femoral tracking pain (kneecap out of alignment on the track of the thigh bone), which causes pain at the front of the knee, particularly when going down stairs.

Although the causes of the RSIs on the job and in sports may in some cases be different from the causes in the person with PPS, the injuries to anatomical structures are similar. Effective treatments of RSIs exist in sports and the workplace; effective treatment modifications for the RSIs of the polio survivor also exist.

Obtain a Specific Anatomic Diagnosis

The most important part of the treatment of RSIs begins with an anatomic diagnosis of the joints, ligaments, muscles, tendons, and/or nerves that are injured. In addition, an activity diagnosis to find out the cause of the injury is important. If the cause is not found and eliminated, or at least modified, treatment will be of little value. The following lists some of the procedures that may be used to make the anatomic and activity diagnoses of RSIs:

- Taking a careful history of the pain including when it started, what activities make it worse, what decreases the pain, and the effect of bedrest on the pain.

- Checking all the joint motions of the area for full or limited range, and for pain or pain-free ranges of motion.
- Testing all muscles for strength and pain-free length.
- Stressing ligaments (stretch lightly) for pain or absence of pain and for pain-free motion.
- Palpating (explore by touching) the area for pain and absence of pain.
- Testing for sensory nerve changes.
- Testing muscle reflexes such as tapping the knee.
- Taking an activity history to determine the cause of injury.

Health professionals whose training prepares them to make the anatomic diagnoses of RSIs include orthopedists, physiatrists, neurologists, and physical therapists specializing in orthopedic and sports physical therapy. Most physicians are not trained to make such a definitive musculoskeletal diagnosis and prefer to refer post-polio survivors to physical therapists or other physicians for specific evaluation. Physical and occupational therapists are trained to evaluate activities of daily living and work performance. They are good resources for helping the survivor determine the activity causing the RSI and alternative ways to avoid the trauma of the activity.

Treatment Principles

Post-polio survivors respond very well to the teaching method of treatment where the therapist serves as an evaluator and a teacher or coach. This model is successful because most people with PPS know their bodies and its capabilities. These survivors are exercise-oriented and highly motivated to improve their situation. For most RSIs the therapist requires only two sessions to four sessions to evaluate and teach the treatment procedures to the survivor and the family member. Periodic reevaluations are necessary to check progress, make corrections or upgrade the exercises and functional activities.

The following sections discuss some of the treatment principles for polio survivors dealing with PPS symptoms. Most patients are already aware of these principles, but some discussion is presented here for review and possibly for new information. These principles include: the RICE principle; rest for the injured part; decreasing inflammation and pain; maintaining and increasing pain-free motions in injured joints; stretching, strengthening, and stabilizing; and making lifestyle changes.

The RICE Principle (Rest, Ice, Compression, and Elevation)

The RICE principle is used in acute athletic injuries and is valuable in the home treatment of RSIs. Rest and cold packs are used extensively; compression is used in acute injuries; and elevation is used for injuries to the extremities, particularly the feet and hands.

Rest the Injured Part

For an injured part, the activity causing the injury needs to be stopped at least temporarily so that tissues may heal. Bedrest is not a good option for the person with PPS if it can be avoided. Rather, the functions of the injured part need to be performed in a different manner. Unfortunately, the survivor may not have any more compensation available to perform the actions of the injured part. It becomes necessary to look to mechanical, electrical, and electronic means and to other people's help. Thus, the seemingly simple "rest of the injured part" can become the major aspect of the treatment. On the other hand, removing the cause of the injury may be all the treatment needed. The activity inventory and its updating are important to help diagnose the cause of the injury.

Decrease Inflammation and Pain (Prevent or Decrease Swelling)

Both heat and cold have anesthetic effects on the body. They relieve pain at the time of treatment. Heat, however, increases inflammation, swelling, and further tissue damage. The pain becomes worse later. Cold, on the other hand, decreases inflammation, swelling, and further tissue damage. Pain relief lasts well beyond the time of application. Nonsteroidal anti-inflammatory drugs (NSAIDs, such as Advil® (or ibuprofen) in combination with cold packs increase effectiveness in decreasing pain. (NSAIDs are prescribed only if appropriate for the individual.) Cold packs can be used anywhere from three to ten times a day, depending on the severity of the pain. They can be very painful if placed directly on a bone and should have one layer of cloth between the pack and the skin. Family packs of frozen peas are an inexpensive substitute for the large packs needed for the back and SIJ.

Maintain and Increase Pain-Free Motions in Injured Joints

Painless repetitive motions of joints improve joint nutrition and help maintain joint range-of-motion. The physical therapist has many ways to unload joints so the individual can perform a pain-free exercise. For example, if a person sits in an office chair with wheels, rests the hands on the table, and then moves back and forth using the feet, he or she will receive passive motion (no muscle activity) to the elbows and shoulders. This exercise would be useful to a person with a shoulder injury who could not raise the arm because of pain. This same exercise can provide pain-free passive motion to the knee. The subject lets the legs and feet rest on the floor and then pushes away and pulls back from the table with the arms. In addition, a simple home pulley system can be set up to provide passive joint range-of-motion using a good arm or leg to pull the injured extremity up and down.

Stretch, Strengthen and Stabilize as Appropriate

The physical therapist has a wide variety of exercises to release tight fascia, mobilize joint surfaces, provide home traction, stretch muscles, release trigger points, massage soft tissues, strengthen or relax muscles, provide joint unloading exercises, and stabilize joint structures. Stretching and strengthening muscles are familiar exercises to people with PPS. At this stage, attempts at stretching or surgically lengthening muscles need to be carefully evaluated because the tightness may have developed to provide stability. For example, often weak calf muscles became tight to provide ankle stability in standing and walking. Release of these muscle tendons causes a collapse of the leg on the foot when walking. Attempting to strengthen muscles to help stabilize joints is of little help because most of the muscles of the person with PPS have achieved maximum strength.

Stabilization of joints is an important function of both muscles and ligaments. When the muscles are weak and the ligaments are overstretched, joint instability and pain occur. While the pain can be treated with cold packs and joint rest, renewal of activity usually requires some form of stabilization. This stabilization is difficult but critical. Stabilization of joints is usually done by taping, orthotics (braces), external supports (SIJ belts), assistive devices, and muscle strengthening (limited).

Make Lifestyle Changes to Prevent Recurrence of Injury

Many problems require minimal changes in lifestyle; some require major changes. An example is the shoulder injury in a person who walks with crutches. Shoulders are not structurally capable of bearing body weight for 30 years, and they do not hold up well. To preserve the ability to walk short distances in the home or at work, this person may need to use a motorized cart for distance locomotion.

In addition to trying to prevent recurrence of the injury, it is helpful to have an immediate treatment plan ready in case reinjury occurs. Immediate application of the RICE principle for acute athletic injury can markedly reduce the extent of the injury and pain. If the RICE principle is applied soon enough, the pain can often be aborted. If the pain continues, it may be time to get in touch with the therapist and ask for help. The manual wheelchair is not a good option because propelling it also leads to RSIs in the upper extremities and to muscle exhaustion if the upper extremities have had any polio involvement.

Treatment Examples

The following paragraphs provide examples of treatment options for polio survivors who are experiencing PPS symptoms. Three musculoskeletal problems are discussed and the home program is presented. Areas described include patello-femoral tracking pain, shoulder subluxation and shoulder blade instability, and sacroileitis.

Patello-femoral tracking pain is an alignment problem of the kneecap caused by imbalance of the quadriceps muscle (on the front of the thigh) when it contracts to straighten the knee. In time, this imbalance causes wear and tear on the underside of the kneecap and the guiding track on the thigh bone (femur). The pain can be so sudden and severe that a fall may occur. Treatment begins with the review by the therapist and survivor of the activities causing the pain. Recommendations may be made to avoid stairs, low chairs, squatting and kneeling, and to use cold packs on the knee to relieve pain and inflammation.

The therapist then shows the survivor and a family member the incorrect motions of the kneecap and how to tape it to correct its line of pull. This treatment requires special taping materials to protect the skin and apply corrective forces to the kneecap. The survivor needs to tape the knee every morning and remove the taping at bedtime. In about a week, the survivor should return to the therapist for a checkup on taping and to receive exercises to reeducate the quadriceps muscle. The problem is usually corrected in one month or two months and the survivor can discontinue the taping. (These special tapes can be obtained in patello-femoral taping kits from rehabilitation product catalogues and stores.)

To prevent recurrence, it is a good idea to use elevators, if possible; elevate some chairs and the commode at home; and, in general, avoid activities that stress the knees. This knee pain is a problem that usually can be corrected and managed in two or a maximum of three therapy visits. The pain may recur, but prompt action using cold packs, taping, and exercises will usually correct the condition. If not, consideration should be given to more stabilization, such as an elasticized knee sleeve with kneecap control.

For shoulder subluxation and shoulder blade instability, taping materials are also effective in relieving the pain of a subluxed shoulder (muscle paralysis around the shoulder with overstretching of ligaments) and in stabilizing a shoulder blade with muscle weakness or paralysis. This problem can be appreciated when one realizes that the shoulder blade is stabilized by 15 different muscles. If just one muscle is weak and cannot function, the stronger ones will overstretch it; therefore, the shoulder blade will not be in the right position for the arm to move. This weakness causes wear and tear, pain, and loss of function in the shoulder. In these instances, taping does not correct the problem; but can prevent the pain during the day while the person is upright and decrease further stretching of the ligaments.

Sacroileitis is one of the most common RSIs in persons with PPS and one of the most difficult to treat. From three to thirty physical therapy visits may be required to help the survivors get to the point of managing their problem. Part of this problem has to do with the inability to totally rest the part. Sideward shifts of the body in walking cause severe abnormal forces on the SIJs. These abnormal forces can be reduced markedly, but not eliminated, by the use of a cane or forearm crutches. Exercises to realign the SIJ and other pelvic bones are complex. A little too much force may result in an overcorrection. Insufficient force leads to undercorrection. Detailed evaluations by the physical therapist are necessary to maintain correction. The main problem is that it is difficult to stabilize the SIJs once the correct position has been achieved. The best stabilization method is the SI belt, which is worn low on the hips. When tightened, the belt compresses and stabilizes the SIJs. The SIJ belts require strong upper extremity strength or assistance from another person to get the needed compression. Regardless of these problems, many survivors have learned to control the pain and dysfunction of their SIJs.

Advantages of Self-Treatment at Home

The teaching method of physical therapy treatment is well-suited to many PPS survivors who have been referred for outpatient or home therapy. It is particularly helpful to those who have limits placed on the amount of physical therapy treatments covered by their medical plans. In this approach, the emphasis is on giving the survivors the responsibility for carrying out the treatment and using the therapist to perform the physical evaluations and teach the specific treatment program. Other advantages are as follows:

- Some aspects of the treatment can be started immediately to relieve pain and inflammation.
- Activities causing the RSI can be decreased or changed right away.
- The survivor avoids the stress, fatigue, and pain of traveling to the therapy facility.
- Treatments can be carried out several times per day at home in contrast to three times a week.
- Polio survivors take responsibility for treatment and care; they usually bring an amazing ingenuity and creativity toward solving the problems.

- Polio survivors learn to take care of their bodies, requiring less and less help from health professionals in the long run.

Limitations of the self-treatment home program include:

- The motivation of the survivors may be limited. While most polio survivors want to take an active role in their treatment, a few are not able to assume this responsibility.
- Family or friend support system is important. In order to participate in the self-treatment program, it is helpful if the survivor has a good support system. Many of the exercises are complex; it may take two to remember all the details or perform the procedure.
- Additional communication between the survivor and the therapist is needed occasionally to answer questions. This interface may be difficult since the therapist has a busy schedule most of the day.
- The teaching method is not comfortable to many physical therapists. Most have been trained to perform hands-on treatment.

SUMMARY

This chapter presents self-treatment principles for persons with PPS. The program requires education of the polio survivors and their families about the nature of the damage caused by the poliovirus to the nerves in the spinal cord and brain, the process of muscle strength recovery, and the effects on the body of long-term overuse of the muscles and joints. With this knowledge and the recommendations and help of health professionals, the survivors can develop a program of lifestyle changes to alleviate the fatigue and pain of PPS and to slow the rate of new muscle weakness. In addition, survivors with and without PPS can learn home treatments to control repetitive stress injuries from abnormal muscle and joint forces.

To begin to decrease the fatigue and muscle pain of PPS takes about a month and should be well under way after three months of resting and making lifestyle changes. However, those who are totally exhausted may take up to a year to make significant improvement. This program is difficult as it often means changing an activity that the survivor worked very hard to accomplish or avoid (such as handicapped parking). The survivor not only needs help but also, more importantly, understanding from family, friends, and colleagues. When the symptoms of PPS became more severe, many people let their world become smaller as they declined to participate in family activities and social events. With a new self-treatment program, they can become animated and excited about their lifestyle changes and the new activities they are now permitted. After the pain and fatigue are gone, activities can be increased slowly to determine limits.

If just a small increase in some activity causes problems, it is an indication that there is no reserve capacity. Further rest and energy conservation are needed to rebuild and restore one's reserve capacity, permitting the survivor the ability to handle an unexpected activity and resume living a fuller life.

7

Psychosocial Dimensions of Polio and Post-Polio Syndrome

RHODA OLKIN

A friend who, like me, had polio once said to me: "FDR delivered the country from the Depression and saved the free world from the Nazis. What have *you* done lately?" While said in jest, the underlying message affects people with polio: We were the rehabilitation success stories. We could be anything, even president of the United States. Well, I'm exhausted just thinking about it.

I had polio in 1954 when I was 15 months old. (I'll do the math for you; I'm 45 years old now.) I contracted polio about a year before the vaccine became available. The primary effects I experienced were on one leg, which is over two inches shorter than the other leg, and mostly paralyzed below the thigh. As a kid, I wore braces of varying lengths on that affected leg and had two major surgeries to correct problems caused by polio. About ten years ago, I began using a scooter (at work or shopping), crutches (shorter distances), or no aid (at home). I consider myself as having post-polio syndrome (PPS), an upsurge in fatigue, weakness, and pain, beginning in my mid-thirties (just in time for me to be a new parent!).

As a polio survivor, a person with PPS, and as a psychologist specializing in disability and family issues, I've had many occasions to think and write about disability. What follows are some of the key points affecting persons with disabilities; some are exclusive to persons with polio/PPS. This chapter covers a lot of territory because the psychological and social implications of polio are broad. The material will be discussed under two main ideas: issues of identity—

how we see ourselves as persons with polio/PPS; and social effects—how we interact with the world and, perhaps more importantly, how the world perceives us.

ISSUES OF IDENTITY

How do we as persons with polio think about and see ourselves? How are we viewed by others? Society casts people with disabilities into various roles. In fact, disability is often called a "social construct," meaning that the disability is best understood in terms of how society perceives disability. Historically, society has perceived disability in three main ways: the moral, medical, and minority models. Each has a perspective on what "the problem" of disability is, who holds the problem, and what are the best avenues to address the problem.

The Moral Model

The moral model is the first and oldest. In this view, disability is a defect caused by moral lapses or sins. It brings shame to the person with the disability and his or her family. They carry the blame for causing the disability. Disability represents divine retribution, failure of faith, moral lapse, or test of faith. The idea that "God gives us only that which we can bear" is prevalent here. In this view, the family of the person with the disability somehow has been selected for its various attributes (faith or strength, or a test thereof). For example, a current mail-order catalogue offered a "Gaelic blessing plaque" with the following message: "May those who love us, love us. And those that don't love us, may God turn their hearts; and if he doesn't turn their hearts, may he turn their ankles so we'll know them by their limping." We see in this saying the moral model view that outward signs of disability reflect inner evils. To those of us who limp, this Gaelic "blessing" is more like a curse. Although the moral model is the oldest view of disability it is still very much in existence; in some cultures, it is the most common view.

The Medical Model

The medical model began in the mid-1800s as medicine became more enlightened and humane. This perspective puts the person with the disability in the role of a patient who has a medical problem. The disability is a defect in, or failure of, a bodily system and, as such, is inherently abnormal and pathological. The goals of intervention are cure, treatment of the physical condition to the greatest extent possible, and rehabilitation, that is, the adjustment of the person with the disability to the condition and the environment. In the United States, the medical model predominates.

The Minority Model

The minority model gets its name from the view that persons with disabilities are a minority group, in the same way that persons of color are a minority group, and one that has been denied its civil rights, equal access, and protection. This model presents a new perspective on disability. It holds that disability is what we say it is. The minority model says that the problem of disability lies not within persons with disabilities, but in the environment that fails to accommodate them and in the negative attitudes of people without disabilities. Key impediments for any minority group are prejudice and discrimination; these impediments also are seen as major problems for those with disabilities. In fact, persons with disabilities often point to social barriers and negative attitudes of others as being among their main problems. This fact means that persons with disabilities have an extra task: they must manage not only the disability, but also others' responses to the disability.

How we define a problem directs our search for solutions. The *moral* model defines the problem as one of sin and moral lapse; therefore, solutions to the curse of disability are to be found through faith, forbearance, exorcism, ostracism, and even death. The *medical* model views the problem as located in the individual; the solutions are medical intervention, aid in adjustment to disability, and modifications of the disabled person's lifestyle. The *minority* model takes the problem out of the realm of the person with a disability and places it in the social, political, and economic world. Solutions include education of those without disabilities about persons with disabilities, laws ensuring equal access and protection and better enforcement of such laws, and increased physical accessibility. It also maintains that decision-making *about* persons with disabilities should be *by* persons with disabilities.

Let me give an example of how the minority model reframes the question and, hence, offers different solutions. Often at work I've been asked whether I will be attending specific events. The unasked question is, "Do we need to pick a place that's physically accessible?" My response is that it doesn't matter whether I will be attending or not. In either case, the site must be accessible. Irrespective of my attendance, there is a compelling moral reason why a site must be accessible. To bring this point home to faculty, I have asked them this question: "Would you hold this function at a site that didn't allow Jews? Would it be relevant to that decision whether someone Jewish was actually in attendance or not?" This question reframes the problem as what it really is, namely a civil rights issue. When we reframe the question in this way, an immediate shift of perspective happens. We now focus on the environment, not on me, the person with the disability: "Will *you* be attending? Can *you* manage two stairs? Do *you* need an extra wide parking space?" Now it becomes the responsibility of the external world to make itself accessible. We translate, "You can't climb stairs," to "Why isn't there a ramp?" We could focus on the faculty and ask the question: "Why is the faculty holding its meeting in a place that is not accessible?" We could focus on the community and ask, "Why was this building erected without due consideration of accessibility for persons with disabilities?" We could also focus on the sociopolitical arena and ask, "Why do we tolerate discrimination against our citizens?" and "At what cost do we do so?" The essential aspect of the minority model is a shift in focus from personal and individual to a focus on the group, environment, attitudes, and discrimination. The problem is not that we are defective; the problem is that we are oppressed.

How you think about yourself as a person with a disability will affect greatly how you think about yourself overall. You may not even be aware that you have a model of disability. Take a few moments to ask yourself some questions that can help bring your model to light. Use the questions in Table 7.1. Some persons may find themselves answering yes to questions in one model that seems to fit them best. Others might find they hold beliefs from more than one model. What

Table 7.1 What Is Your Model of Disability?

Model	Questions to Ask Yourself
MORAL MODEL	■ Do you feel shame or embarrassment about your disability? ■ Do you feel you bring dishonor to the family? ■ Do you try to hide and minimize the disability as much as possible? ■ Do you try to make as few demands on others as possible, because it's *your* problem and hence *your* responsibility? ■ Do you try to make your disability inconspicuous? ■ Do you think your disability is a test of your faith, or as a way for you to prove your faith? ■ Do you think your disability is a punishment for you or your family's failings?
MEDICAL MODEL	■ Compared to FDR's time, do you think that life for persons with disabilities has improved tremendously? ■ Do you think even FDR wouldn't have to hide his disability today? ■ Do you try to make as few demands on others as possible, because you think you should be able to find a way to do it yourself? ■ Do you dress in ways that maximize your positive features and minimize the visibility of the disability? ■ Do you believe that the major goals of research should be to prevent disabilities and find cures for those who already have disabilities? ■ Do you think that persons with disabilities do best when they are fully integrated into the nondisabled community?
MINORITY MODEL	■ Do you identify yourself as part of a minority group of persons with disabilities? ■ Do you feel kinship and belonging with other persons with disabilities? ■ Do you think that not enough is being done to assure rights of persons with disabilities? ■ When policies and legislation are new do you evaluate them in terms of their effects on persons with disabilities? ■ Do you think the major goals of research should be to improve the lives of persons with disabilities by changing policies, procedures, funding, and laws? ■ Do you think that persons with disabilities do best when they are free to associate in both the disabled and nondisabled communities, as bicultural people?

is important is not where you fit but where you feel most at home, what works for you, and what allows you the greatest degree of satisfaction and contentment with yourself and others. However, some of you may find you fit into a model and wish you didn't. Your fit is uncomfortable or it arouses feelings of anxiety, anger, or sadness. This reaction is not unusual. Keep several things in mind. First, there is no such thing as complete adjustment to disability. You're never *there*; you're only *traveling* there. Thus, your thoughts about disability will constantly change and evolve. Second, the development of PPS symptoms means a whole new trunk-full of disability stuff to unload. Feelings you thought you'd already dealt with may reemerge. However, any discomfort with the model you're currently experiencing is a positive sign that you are not sweeping the disability issues under the rug. By recognizing your feelings you leave open more of an opportunity to change them. You must do two things for yourself. One is to talk to other people with polio/PPS. The other is to ease up on yourself. For now, you feel what you feel; but this too shall pass.

Being Bicultural

According to the minority model, some experiences are shared by all persons with disabilities, such as stereotyping, prejudice, and discrimination. Thus you belong to a community of persons with disabilities. You may not think of yourself as a person with a disability, and you may not identify with other people with disabilities. Regardless of how you see yourself, you are a part of a minority group, that is, persons with disabilities. But you also belong in another community, that of your family, friends, and neighborhood. This community is mostly or even all nondisabled. Thus you are bicultural, living with a disability in the nondisabled world. Many of you are at least tricultural, as there are many other communities and groups to which you might belong. Some of you will identify and affiliate more with one group than the other; some will feel torn between them; and still others will feel exclusively a part of one camp, mostly oblivious to the other. Again, as in finding your model of disability, what matters is how well it works for you and your family. If you can remain open to both cultures more options become available to you, with two sets of role models, influences, and assets.

Updating Your Diagnosis

Those of us with polio got used to thinking of ourselves as *post*-polio. We weathered its acute onset, and then we proceeded to carry on to the best of our abilities. The prevailing motto was, "Use it or lose it." Use it we did. We were taught to push ourselves, not to impose or accept limits. We got caught up in the exercise era whose slogan was, "No pain, no gain." We experienced pain, but we persevered. Then suddenly, after a lifetime of messages that we could be anything, do anything we set our minds to, that there were no limits—after all that—we learned we had a new diagnosis: post-polio syndrome. Now the motto became, "Conserve it to preserve it." Suddenly we were told to moderate our activities, develop a new lifestyle, conserve energy. Wasn't that a whack in the head? Living with polio now required a readjustment of identity from a person who *had* polio to a person who *has* PPS. Becoming *more* of a minority member is not something that happens in other minority groups; you generally don't get more Jewish, more Vietnamese, or more Hispanic. This feature of getting more disabled means we have the task of constantly adjusting, and then when we think we've adjusted, we have to adjust again.

This change in our disabilities affected not only us but also our families. Our parents may have felt a reawakening of some of their earlier feelings about our contracting polio. Our spouses and partners may have had to readjust their thinking and participate in altering lifestyles to accommodate new losses. For those with children still in the home, or who became new parents, the combined demands of childrearing and disability had to be managed.

One effect of new symptoms and needs was that many of us had to be strong self-advocates. We had to find doctors knowledgeable about polio and gain access to them in this time of managed care. We had to adjust our activities and our lifestyles, renegotiate job descriptions, find new ways to accomplish tasks, learn about assistive technologies, and acquire new skills. Most of us were children or young adults when we incurred polio, and our parents were our advocates. Now we had to take the role back, usually without any specific training, modeling, or guidance, on how best to become our own advocates. It was on-the-job training. For example, I became an expert on scooters and insurance rules for obtaining durable medical equipment. I found jar openers, spring-loaded scissors, grabbers, electronic lamp switches that allow me to turn off the light from bed, and other labor-saving devices. At work, I had to get an elevator installed, find handicapped parking near my office, move a doorway to lessen hallway obstruction, and effect many other accommodations. In every sphere of my life, changes were needed, ranging from small (a device to hold bagels while I sliced them) to large (a new van, scooter, and lift that would all work together). Some were necessitated by newer PPS symptoms (e.g., a different keyboard for the computer); others were extensions of older long-term needs (finding shoemakers to correctly alter my shoes); and others were specific to particular life tasks (finding someone to attach a child seat to the back of my scooter). In all cases, I had to advocate for myself, know my rights, and feel confident in pursuing them. Instead I felt overwhelmed.

This previous list of accomplishments represents a full *decade* of work. Often I did nothing. Many times my husband shouldered much of the responsibility of getting something done. Other times I made do. The main lesson is this: Tackle *one* thing at a time. Always. The list of tasks above may seem impressive, but your list too will add up over time. It's vital to keep a perspective on what's essential (mobility); what makes life easier (new curb cut), reduces pain (better desk chair), or fatigue (closer light switch); and what's nice (bagel holder). None of us signed up for the job of advocate, but it comes with the territory. However, as we take the time to make our lives easier, we must be mindful of our overall load. If you're embarking on a fight with your insurance company, don't tackle getting the city to install a curb cut at the same time, and, by all means, give up a little on the need for a clean kitchen floor!

SOCIAL INTERACTIONS AS A PERSON WITH A DISABILITY

If disability is a social construct, what are the *rules* of disability? I believe these are most apparent with regard to feelings. The role of a person with a disability is defined in part by ideas of what we must and must not feel. This definition is particularly apparent with regard to cheerfulness (encouraged), anger (prohibited), and mourning (required). Additionally, disability has effects on one's privacy, personal power and control.

Regulation of Mood

The requirement to regulate mood is a common part of disability. The dual requirement exists of what to be and what not to be: one must be cheerful; one must not be angry. This issue of forced cheerfulness has been addressed most eloquently in Hugh Gallagher's *FDR's Splendid Deception*. FDR, a president with a profound disability, successfully hid the extent of his disability from the world. He was the embodiment of the bargain between persons with disabilities and America: "We (the non-disabled) will let you (the disabled) live and work among us, provided that you never make us too aware of your disability or its attendant difficulties, and that you at all times appear cheerful." We have been unable to break free of this bargain. We see it evidenced in a 1993 obituary in the newspaper of a major city. At the top of the obituary is a picture of an attractive young woman. The caption has her name, and in smaller letters says, "She was paralyzed in 1985." Her paralysis is her main identity. The title of the obituary is, "Radio career cut by gunman's bullet." This model and disk jockey had to switch careers when she became paralyzed by ". . . a gunman's bullet on a deserted highway in 1985." She died of breathing problems related to double pneumonia, but this 28-year-old woman will be remembered ". . . as a fighter who overcame the obstacles that paralysis put in her way and managed to live a happy and full life." Note how the obstacles stem from her paralysis (the medical model) not from an inaccessible environment (minority model). Also, we see the notion that persons with disabilities will not be happy unless they overcome the disability and *manage* to have a full life. A quote from a friend takes this theme over the top: "She never complained. She'd always have this big smile." Just like the image of FDR sitting behind a desk, his head thrown back, a huge grin on his face, and in one hand, the cigarette in its long holder. Forty years later, we have this young woman who "always" had this big smile. Disabled people are supposed to smile. In case we missed this point, the latest reminder comes from, of all places, Mattel toys. Mattel announced in May of

1997 that it is issuing the first Barbie (actually, friend of Barbie) in a wheelchair. They've decided to name her "Share-a-smile Becky."

The flip side of the requirement of cheerfulness is the rule against anger. Persons with disabilities are not supposed to be angry. If we are, it is hard for others to accept or understand. The problem is that we are seen as being angry in response to a single event. Often the anger is not about one event, but about a history of similar events. Without awareness of this history, it looks as if we're overreacting, and this is seen as indicative of a lack of adjustment. Anger also suggests that we are not grateful enough. We, who depend to some extent on the assistance of others, cannot express anger because to do so would jeopardize our continued care. Onset of PPS symptoms, however, may have put many of us over a just-noticeable threshold, such that we tire more easily, experience pain more frequently, and have less energy readily available. In other words, we could use a little more help. We must not complain and must request help graciously and cheerfully. We agree to this attitude in part because we want others to do things for us because they like us rather than because they pity us. We *should* be grateful not only for others' assistance, but also because we are so much better off than others with worse disabilities—able-bodied people can look me in the eye and make this statement, unaware of the irony. Like the big fish eating the littler fish eating the littler fish, we are always supposed to compare ourselves to the smaller fish, not the next larger fish in the chain. By keeping us grateful not to be an even smaller fish (i.e., more disabled), those without disabilities protect themselves from our envy and resentment. The problem of anger is also seen in rules about how others should act toward us. Just as we are not supposed to get angry at others, others are not supposed to get angry at us. Perhaps others see the visible sign of disability as implying a deeper inner weakness, a basic flaw, such that anger toward us would destroy us.

The common perspective on the "psychology of disability" is that it represents a loss—a loss of the healthy or undamaged body, a loss of function. As such, the loss *must* be mourned before the process of *adjustment* can be accomplished. The problem is that not all people with disabilities mourn. Although in many instances persons who sustain a disability's onset or exacerbation may well experience a period of mourning (sadness, loss, and grieving), this feeling is not inevitable or universal. If we are not mourning, others tend to think of us as somehow superhuman. The logic goes as follows: "You have a disability. Having a disability is awful. Therefore you must be suffering. I see you as suffering." If the evidence overwhelmingly indicates that the person with the disability is not suffering, the other then thinks: "You are not suffering in a situation in which suffering should occur. Why not? It must be because you are brave, courageous, plucky, extraordinary, superhuman." Those are the choices: suffering, loss and mourning, or continual pluckiness. The person with a disability who fails to conform to these requirements has a "bad attitude."

For the person with a disability, the latitude for a normal range of emotions is curtailed. We are expected never to let the disability get us down. Virtually all persons with disabilities have been told how brave they were, sometimes for *simply getting up in the morning*. At the same time people—even family who presumably know the family member with the disability well—overestimate the misfortune and suffering of persons with disabilities. Many people assume that there are higher levels of distress, anxiety, and depression among persons with disabilities; but people with disabilities are more like people without disabilities than unlike them. There is no *polio profile*. (Well, except for the fact that we're superior people!)

Given these rules about mood for people with disabilities, it might be good to pause and consider how they have affected us. Have you restricted your options of different feelings? Are you free to feel anger and to express it? Do you believe that as PPS symptoms increase, you must mourn? When someone you don't know asks, "What happened to you?", what is your internal response? What is your external response? Remember that one theme here is that what you feel is okay; otherwise, this chapter would just be another imposition on your feelings. However, you do not need to suffer needlessly with a treatable depression or anxiety disorder. (See Chapter Eight.)

The disabled community has a unique feature. It is a community with open enrollment; anyone can join at any time by acquiring a disability. This fact contributes to some able-bodied peoples' need to distance themselves from us, from the knowledge that this, too, could happen to *them*. This knowledge may spur people to find reasons why it couldn't happen to them; such a reason is provided by holding the person with the disability at fault for the condition. Polio has been less subject to this view in that polio was widely perceived as a random event, not the fault of the patient. But as time goes on, more people look at me quizzically, wondering if my parents perhaps failed to get me vaccinated. If the polio can be *explained*, it bolsters other peoples' feelings of protection and immunity from disability.

Privacy and Control

Being a person with a visible disability is to be stripped of many of the usual boundaries of self. Because a part of oneself (one's disability status) is apparent to others, one becomes a person who can be approached at will. A somewhat analogous situation is when a woman is in the third trimester of pregnancy. Acquaintances feel free to ask personal questions ("What are you hoping for, a boy or a girl?" "Was this a planned pregnancy?"). Indeed, perfect strangers come up and pat your belly as if your stomach had pushed through and broken that invisible shield around your personal space. Something about the state of visible pregnancy invites such intrusions. These same kinds of intrusions happen with disability as well—the personal questions, the intrusive touching. The exposure makes one subject to conversations strangers may feel free to strike up, questions they feel free to ask, curiosity they feel free to express about your condition. These invasions happen unpredictably, intruding into your day unbidden. Let me describe one example. I get off my scooter in a shoe store to examine something more closely. A man sitting and waiting his turn sees me able to walk and says to me, "Good for you!" and punches the air in front of him enthusiastically. He feels free to comment on my behavior. Suddenly I stand there not as a woman buying shoes, but as a person with a disability, the fact of my disablement a blinking neon sign. This can happen anytime, anywhere. It can happen once a week or twice in ten minutes. It can happen in front of my children, who will learn through repetitions of this scenario that something is wrong with having a mother with a disability.

With this blinking neon sign on me, it's hard to be invisible or just one of the crowd. When I come late to a meeting, *everyone* knows it. Having a visible disability means always being noticed, standing out, being different, *everywhere you go*. People will respond to your differentness, and not just to themselves—they respond in a way that forces their response on you. Some will want to heal you (embrace their religion and throw away your crutches); some offer redemption (Jesus loves you). But many need to tell you how really okay they are with you as you are, and in so doing, prove the opposite. Sometimes you just want to be left alone, anonymous, invisible, just once.

Paradoxically, given how visible I generally am, at times I am completely invisible. Sometimes when people meet me for the first time, I'm on my scooter. If at the second meeting, I am walking (on crutches or unaided), many times people simply don't recognize me. They think we've never met. I got stored in their memories as a scooter, and they sure would remember a scooter if they saw it again. But they don't see *me*. One year my son's teacher, having met me on my scooter, kept trying to clarify at our second meeting (I was on foot) exactly what my relationship to my son was. I finally understood her confusion, and said "I'm his mother." (Not the scooter; me.)

Often people make comments about the nature of the disability itself. Someone might say to me, "I saw you walking in the store the other day; you seem to be doing better." (In fact, this statement is complete fantasy on his or her part.) I could explain. I could say that one doesn't get better at this stage post-polio and, in fact, gets worse with aging and PPS, that I always walk in that particular store because it's too crowded for my scooter, but I don't. He or she doesn't know me that well. I don't want to have this conversation with that person. I will take all the time needed to answer the questions of a child; if you are a friend of mine, ask me anything. It's not that I'm *oversensitive* about my disability. It's just that I don't want to share personal information with strangers any more than anyone else does.

People want to let you know that you're not the first of *your kind* they've met. Just as the pregnant woman incurs stories of others' childbirth experiences (just what you don't want to hear), the person with a disability engenders stories of other persons with disabilities. ("My uncle had a disability.") How is one to respond to this? Here the issues of privacy and regulation of mood collide. Get angry, and it will be seen as *your* problem, that you have a chip on your shoulder. Plus, you are seen as representing your group, giving a worse name to persons with disabilities. If you ignore these remarks, it can be like an insidious bacterium invading your immune system. You could explain to the other person the effect of the remark on you, but really, when did you sign up for this career of disability educator to the world? So you say, "Oh really," in as disinterested a voice as you can muster, or try to joke, "Funny, you don't look like the nephew of a person with a disability." No matter how you respond you are likely to enter the next encounter just a little more warily and be a little *overreactive* to the next person who tells you about an uncle with a disability.

All of these intrusions into one's privacy contribute to a sense of loss of control. The invasions of privacy occur at others' whims. They affect not only the person with a disability, but also his or her family. You possess information about your disability ("I had polio"; "I can't walk that distance"), but you have control over this information only as long as you tell no one. Once the information is revealed, you lose control of the information, which then may be shared, misrepresented, recorded, gossiped about, etc.

A further factor in loss of control is that polio is not a stable disorder as once thought. As we begin to experience PPS symptoms, it becomes clear that the future course of polio/PPS is unpredictable. Part of our task is to learn to live with this unpredictability. I have seen persons with disabilities respond to these demands of disability and uncertainty in a variety of ways. In a testament to human resiliency and resourcefulness, there are many versions of making it work.

The Disability Experience

Disability leads to certain kinds of experiences, and these experiences in turn influence and shape the world view of the person with a disability. One experience is the attitudes of others toward disability, as discussed earlier. There are other commonalities of disability experience. These experiences are partly personal—i.e., the things that happen to oneself—but also events that happen to others with disabilities, events to which one resonates. This disability experience shapes one's perceptions of, and stance toward, the world.

Let me give an example, showing how disability can become the framer of one's world view on a subject. About eight months after the birth of my son, he and I went to the grocery store. I came back to my car with the baby and a full cart of groceries. I took my son up into my arms, and as I was opening the trunk, a woman stopped and said, "May I help you?" I gratefully accepted. To my amazement, she forcefully took my son out of my arms (possibly intending that she hold him while I loaded the groceries—the opposite of what I'd assumed she'd offered). Both he and I freaked, and I took my crying son back. The woman turned to walk away, saying, "I know, I know, *you people* like to do it all yourselves." This emotionally powerful incident might have remained an isolated one, but within the next few years I read of the Tiffany Callo case (which I remember as the case of a mother with a disability losing custody of her baby). I also read an account of a Michigan case of two parents with disabilities who used personal attendants and lost custody of their child because they were unable to care for him without assistance. Then I saw an article in a scholarly journal that stated that disabled women were at greater risk for losing child custody. Thus, I had four events that helped shape my view—one personal experience, and three events I read about that had personal meaning for me—that I, as a mother with a disability, could lose my child more easily than a mother without a disability.

This example shows how my perspective was shaped in one area. Suppose this process were repeated over many areas, as indeed it has been. Soon much of my perspective is influenced by my experiences as a person with a disability. In other words, it doesn't take many experiences or events to profoundly shape my world view. Even if 99 percent of my experiences are positive, the one percent of negative experiences can have a greater impact, if they are emotionally evocative, personally meaningful, powerful, and I have reason to believe that they are not isolated instances (e.g., by reading that they have happened to others). Soon my *reality* becomes different from those of people without disabilities. This perception is why your bicultural status is so important. You have a group of people who do understand because their perspective has been shaped similarly to yours. So many people describe discovering the disabled community as *coming home*, precisely because of this wealth of shared experiences. This statement is not meant to minimize some of the emotional difficulties of identifying yourself with a group of people with disabilities. When I first walked into a room full of people in wheelchairs, little people, people using sign language, those with helper dogs or white canes, I thought, "I'm not one of them. I had polio, but they're *disabled.*" It took awhile to sense how comfortable this group was for me, how so much that went unsaid was understood.

There is a second way that disability shapes perspective. We had a negative event in our lives—we contracted polio. The occurrence of this event, the fact of its having happened, taught us that lightning can strike. For some people, this knowledge influences how subsequent events are viewed. For instance, I worried about having amniocentesis during pregnancy because of the risk of miscarriage. I was assured that the risk was very low and told statistics which I didn't find in the least bit reassuring. Why not? Because in 1954 only two people in the state of Michigan contracted polio, and I was one of them. Those odds were minuscule, but they happened. It was a lesson to me in another way: I knew that many other people had not learned that lightning could strike them, and I both envied and disliked them for this. And in an odd way, I felt I had special knowledge and prized this specialness.

I feel *special* in other ways as well. In hundreds of ways throughout my week, I do things differently from nondisabled people. I park in designated areas. I enter through different doors to avoid stairs or heavy doors. I can't use the bathroom in one store because it's inaccessible, but I can use the restroom next door because the owner makes an exception for me; I don't go to a particular theater that has stairs. Salesclerks in my local stores and neighbors along my route to the stores all remember me; I'm the lady on the scooter.

I have some special skills related to my disability. First, I can identify fine gradations of pain, knowing when the pain crosses the line from nuisance to warning signal. From about ten paces away from a curb, I can tell if my right or left foot will be the one to go up (or down) the step, and I can change the length of my pace accordingly. I have well-honed skills in sensing nonverbal responses of others, sharpened by a lifetime of figuring out how people reacted to my disability. I have developed methods of managing stigma. And I know from the pain in my right ankle when the barometer drops and it's likely to rain!

I am not like everyone else. I am the exception. Things don't apply to me. I, and others with disabilities, are constantly the exceptions. We are so used to pushing and shoving our way in, being our own advocates, being on the outskirts, being the exception, being different, that we start to think we are the exception in ways and situations other than those related to the disability.

Role Models, Mentors, and Heroes: Living in a Nondisabled World

If a child is the only one with a disability in the family, to whom does he or she look as a model? What are the norms for people with polio? Where are the role models for parenting with a disability? Who are our icons, our heroes? And who gets to choose: *us* (i.e., persons with disabilities) or *them* (i.e., people without disabilities)?

Television has shown us several models of disability. There have been at least five different roles that persons with disabilities (played by nondisabled actors) have had on TV. One is *Ironsides*, where the moral strength of the main actor was symbolized in the strong steel of his wheelchair. Disability is often used as a metaphor, such as the pretty woman who dates a blind man because she doesn't want to be liked only for her looks; she wants the man to *see* the real her. Another common role is that of the villain with a disability, whose disability explains the villainy (e.g., the psychopathic killer with a clubfoot). A less common figure is the background character, usually in a wheelchair, who has no lines but quietly goes about doing regular work. Only occasionally do we see a well-developed character with depth and multifacets, only one of which is the disability. (Lenny, a man with mental retardation on *LA Law*, comes to mind.) What do we learn from these models of disability? The main lesson is that, just as our feelings have been restricted, we are further hemmed in by a lack of options in role models. Forced to buy off the rack in the back, our clothing selections are limited. We must expand them so that we can find ones that fit us comfortably.

Where else can we look for role models? One problem is that we *do* look to the media for role models, but of course persons in the media are newsworthy in some way. Therefore, many media stories about persons with disabilities simply reinforce the prevailing myths. Sometimes these are stories of the "Can you believe how plucky she is?" variety, profiles of persons with disabilities doing ordinary things but assumed to be extraordinary because they do them with a disability. Other times the stories are of noble endeavors made more heroic because of the disability. An example might be a marathon "runner" who completes the race in a wheelchair. These stories perpetuate *overcoming*—the need to be better than everyone else to be thought of as just as good.

I was not immune to these forces. At 20 years of age, I still thought that I, like FDR, could be president, at least metaphorically. To prove it, I climbed on crutches 3½ miles up a mountain. Being at the top was exhilarating. Climbing down the shorter but steeper route, however, it became clear that there had been a recent rock slide, and the trail was covered by rocks of various sizes. When using crutches, there is a moment of faith in which you raise your feet off the ground and put all your weight on the crutches. As I did this, the crutches would turn out to be on unsteady rocks, and I'd begin to slide down the mountainside. The descent was exhausting and nerve-wracking. My energy already spent, I still had the steepest part ahead of me, and had to negotiate my way down past the falls on the "mist trail"—over a hundred very steep, narrow, wet and slippery steps, between a wall of rock, covered with slippery wet moss, and a waterfall rushing past in a crescendo of water and noise. I made a slow, treacherous, careful descent, while behind me a line of people backed up. I could hear them: "What's the hold up?" "I don't know, something seems to be holding up the line." "There's a girl there on crutches." "What's she doing here?" Well, what a good question. What *was* I doing there?

That trip up the mountain was a watershed event for me, although it took me ten years to realize it. Raised to think I could do anything I set my mind to, I tested the boundaries of "anything" and found that there were limits. This lesson took many more years and trials to learn. I *could* climb a mountain, but I didn't *have* to, and why would I want to, anyway?

Most of us are just regular people. Itzak Perlman was one of my early heroes, in part because he always insisted that his TV appearances show him walking out on stage with his crutches. He said that, when he began playing violin professionally, all the stories about him described him as a man who had polio, and who also played the violin. It was only after he became one of the four premier violinists in the world did the stories switch to describing him as a premier violinist, who also happened to have had polio. Most of us are not premier violinists. Most of us will never climb a mountain. But we would still like to be thought of as people first, not as a disability. When we talk about using "people first" language ("person with a disability" as opposed to "disabled person"), this is what we mean. We want people to look at us and see us, not the disability.

If we don't want people without disabilities to choose our heroes for us, who would we choose? My first role model (I was about seven years old) was a colleague of my father's who also had polio, which left him with considerable weakness and paralysis. I most vividly remember that he didn't have sufficient stomach muscles to produce a decent sneeze. He lived in a two-story house with an inclinator chair—a chair that travels on a rail up and down the stairs. He was married, had children and a career. He lived a *normal* life. It was my first example that people like me could be normal.

The disabled community is full of heroes, people of enormous courage. Many of you are among this group. Having a disability is hard work, yet we do it every day. But must we be mountain-climbers too? We must not focus so much attention on the mountain-climbers that we lose sight of the profoundly ordinary persons with disabilities who are not premier violinists.

8

Polio/Post-Polio Syndrome and Specific Life Tasks

RHODA OLKIN

This chapter integrates a variety of information for persons with polio. It goes beyond the wealth of technical and medical information to focus on issues that allow us not merely to survive but to thrive. Some of these issues touch on our deepest emotions, call for thoughtful reflection, and challenge us to find resolution. The chapter can serve as a roadmap into the future and lead to greater comfort and security. It has two major sections: Families of Persons With Disabilities, and Romance and Dating. Subtopics include assistive technology, self-concept, aging, and matters of sexuality, romance, marriage, pregnancy and childbirth.

FAMILIES OF PERSONS WITH DISABILITIES

Disability is a family affair. You may think of polio as something that happened to *you*, especially if you were quite young at the time and unable to understand how your parents were affected. Of course, the polio was also something that happened to your family, just as post-polio syndrome (PPS) is affecting not only you but also your current family. Any new or worsened symptoms you experience now may reawaken old feelings in both you and your parents. As you struggle to accept the polio in your past and PPS of the present, your family struggles as well. In part, they take their cue from you;

the more accepting you are, the easier it is for them. This is a big responsibility, to have to handle both your own emotions and set the stage for others to handle theirs. We must remember, however, that *accepting* the disability does not mean *liking* it. Let's face it: who needs declining capabilities, increased fatigue, and chronic pain? We knew we had polio in the past, but we didn't know we could develop PPS. Two for the price of one isn't always such a bargain!

Our Parents

When we had polio, few treatments were available (iron lung, hot packs). Our survival was initially uncertain, and the extent of our disabilities unknown. This situation was traumatic for our parents. Many felt guilty—irrationally so; but those of you who are parents know that this is a common reaction when bad things happen to our children. If we were very young, our parents had to decide how to raise us as children with disabilities. If we were older, they had to renegotiate their relationships to us.

Sometimes, the parents and hence the family, remember polio as something that happened to *them*. The story of the polio becomes *their* story. However, *you* "own" the polio. You should have *your* polio story. It can be helpful to go back over the onset with your parents and siblings. Although painful, it can help to hear from each person in the family what the experience was like from his or her perspective. What emerges is that there is not just one polio story, but several. This allows you to have your own story of having polio. You need your own story because now you have to add to it the PPS story. Chances are this PPS story is going to contain many elements of the polio onset story, both for you and your parents. This story is important because what you tell yourself about your disability determines in part how you feel about it. For example, the story I tell of having polio is one of bad luck: there were only two cases in the state of Michigan, and I was one of them. I grew up aware that an unlikely negative event had occurred to me. I never thought, "Why me?" Instead, I thought, "Of course me; I have bad luck." Then when PPS was first being reported in news stories, I thought, "You know that if it happens to anyone, it will happen to me." Thus, my pattern of thought remained constant from the polio to the PPS story.

Seeing the connection between the two helped me realize that my polio and PPS story made me vulnerable to depression. This insight helped motivate me to change the story and take more control over how I live with PPS. As one example, I made my house more physically accessible; I decided not to be disadvantaged in my own home. In this way, I created my own "luck." You can use the tasks listed in Table 8.1 and the questions in Tables 8.2 and 8.3 to help you see how you might use your own story to understand yourself better, and then use that knowledge to help you live with PPS now.

Disability is not like most other minority groups where the whole family is the same minority. Usually the person with the disability is the only one in the family. Therefore, a key source of support and modeling—the family—might not be a help but a hindrance. Whether it was a mother who overprotected you, a father who couldn't discuss it, a sibling who was embarrassed by you, an uncle who babied you, or a parent who worried that no one could ever love you—sometimes our family's stories were not helpful. By creating our own disability stories we outgrow our family in one respect, and this can create discomfort. The discomfort will be reduced if we give up on the idea that the families we grew up in have to agree or change with us; we must agree to disagree. The creation of our own story does not change their story, and we must not insist that it do so.

Because of the time in history when we were born, we came of age and attended school prior to legislation mandating nondiscrimination in education of children with disabilities (Education for All Handicapped Children Act of 1975). The Americans with Disabilities Act wasn't passed until 1990. The minority model of disability was barely starting to take hold, and most people did not think of people with disabilities as members of a minority group. The net result is that we were denied some of our civil rights. We may have become too readily accepting of entering through back doors, not being able to get on the bus. For many of us, our parents were our staunchest advocates. As we take back our own disability stories, we have to take the responsibilities that go with them, including being our own advocates, sometimes for the first time. Living well means retaining control over the course of our own lives. For those of us with PPS, living well also means retaining control over how we handle our disabilities.

Assistive Technology

I am a strong supporter of using assistive devices and technology, ranging from no-tech (a device that breaks the vacuum seal on bottles) to low-tech (a remote control unit to turn lights on/off) to high-tech (voice-activated environmental controls). All of these technologies have the same goal: to enable you to do a task more easily or at all. Sometimes the use of such a device seems more personal, that is, it becomes a part of our self-image. For example, I began using an electric scooter about 10 years ago. This required a change in how I view myself and a more honest acknowledgment of my current level of disability. The change wasn't easy, but after a few years of scooter use, I could see that I could do so much more with much less energy than would otherwise have been possible. In retrospect, it is hard to see how I could have coped with two small children without this assistive technology. The problem is we can't have hindsight beforehand! It is hard to know how much something will help us until we try it, and sometimes we are reluctant to try it because it changes our status or doesn't fit our self-image.

Many parents with disabilities find devices that help them, or they alter a ready-made object. For example, I had a kid's bicycle seat attached to the back of my electric scooter. I thought up the idea on my own, then had to search for someone to do the work for me. Sometimes, we don't know that something is possible so we don't know what to ask for. Picking babies up off the floor, getting the side of the crib down, bathing a slippery baby, and running alongside the two-wheeler your kid is just learning to ride are potentially difficult or impossible tasks. Assistive technologies can make the difference between doing them or not doing them at all, can save the wear and tear on your body and prevent injury, and can help manage your energy expenditures so that you have more available for other things.

For those who feel some reluctance to use devices that seem to make the disability more noticeable, several ways can ease the process. Going to a medical or hospital supply store is a good way to try out equipment for the first time because no one there will think anything of it. I found that I could use the scooter more easily with strangers and family first, and second with good friends. It took much longer to feel comfortable using it with coworkers. In that

Table 8.1 Self-Assessment to Increase Well-being

Task	Goal
Discuss your polio onset with the family you grew up in. Listen for each person's polio story. Become aware of your own polio story. See how this fits with your PPS story.	Use the story to develop strategies for maximizing self-determination.
Examine how you "own" the polio and PPS. In what ways do you take control of living with PPS symptoms, and in what ways do you let things happen, wait for something or someone else to make decisions for you, or for "luck" to decide?	Increase your feelings of control and power in your life. This results in a better sense of well-being.
Assess any symptoms you might have of depression or anxiety. (*See Table 8.2* for a self test on depression.) Remember that everyone feels some sadness and some anxiety, so do not seek to have zero symptoms.	Become aware of any treatable emotional disorder and seek professional assistance. PPS is hard enough without an additional burden of a depression or anxiety disorder.
Take stock of your current roles and functions. (*See Table 8.3* for some questions to ask yourself in making this assessment.)	Achieve greater balance in your life, avoid overdoing and then collapsing; keep a more even level of energy throughout the day and the week.
Ask yourself if there is any possible assistive device or technology that could save labor, make tasks easier, conserve energy. What keeps you from using them? What tasks could be relegated to other people? What tasks can you let go altogether?	It's really true: You must conserve to preserve it.
If you had $500 to spend on your house, what one change would make it easier for you to live there? Consider small changes that save energy. Examples might be building a ramp to the front door, changing doorknobs to bars instead of knobs, finding a lower work surface in the kitchen and leaving a chair there, putting grab bars around tub and shower, making a sliding door self-closing, purchasing a remote control for lights and putting it within easy reach, putting lights on timers.	Don't use energy unnecessarily. Save your energy for more important things, such as your family and friends.

Table 8.1 Self-Assessment to Increase Well-being (Continued)

Task	Goal
Think about the roles and functions in your household (e.g., provider, housekeeper, gardener, childrearing, romantic partner, emotional support). Consider how these are presently divided. Think about which ones must be done by family members (e.g., cuddling the children), which could be shared or taken over by another family member (e.g., washing dishes), which could be hired out (e.g., vacuuming), and which might not need to be done at all now (e.g., putting the last five years of photos into albums).	Use good communication skills in the family to problem-solve how the family will function without overburdening any one person.
Evaluate your family's stressors and resources. Make a list of each, then try to make the stressor list shorter and the resource list longer. Factors to consider might include size of family, size of extended family and how close they live, finances, the life stage of the family e.g., teenagers leaving home for first time is often stressful, as are other times of (transition), changes in job, income, or housing, health of all family members, friendship, divorce, custody arrangements.	A balance between stresses and resources leads to better coping. If stressors outweigh resources the entire family functioning suffers.

setting I try to be seen as a competent person who happens to have a disability; introducing the scooter made the disability more noticeable than I felt comfortable with. Others also may find that using a product at home is easier than in public or at work. It can be helpful to rehearse how to respond to others' comments about the device because such comments are inevitable.

Grab bars, ramps, lowered countertops in the kitchen so you can sit at them, bottle openers—these are small things that help conserve energy, avoid injury, decrease pain, and enable greater independence. This independence is important not just for you, but for your family. Families should be a part of any decision to use assistive devices. This is not to say that these transitions will necessarily be easy. Some of them (e.g., grab bars around the toilet) are relatively private; others (e.g., building a ramp to the front door) are more public; and some (e.g., using a scooter) involve changes in self-

Table 8.2 Questions to Assess Depression and Anxiety

- Feeling sad or blue part of each day, or more often than not.
- Less interest and pleasure in things that were previously enjoyable.
- Difficulty sleeping, or sleeping more than usual.
- Difficulty concentrating or making everyday decisions.
- Weight loss without dieting, or change in appetite.
- Feelings of worthlessness, guilt, or inadequacy in many parts of your life.
- Recurring thoughts of death or suicide.

If you answer yes to three or more of these, you may be suffering from an episode of depression, or you may have a medical condition that is causing these symptoms. Consult your primary care physician.

image. You may have strong feelings about these assistive devices, as may others in your family. Including the family early and throughout transitions increases the likelihood that you actually will use the devices. Further, if you and your family can provide mutual emotional support and encouragement about the assistive technology, technology use will be made more a part of the family's functioning. Only then can your use of assistive technology contribute to the family's well-being.

You and Your Partner

You and your polio/PPS are a package deal. Most of us had polio prior to early adulthood, and thus chose partners who were accepting of us and our disabilities. We chose partners who could love all, not just parts, of us. On the other hand, as our functioning changes,

Table 8.3 Questions to Assess Roles and Functions

- What is your daily and weekly balance between work and play?
- How much time per day and per week do you set aside just for relaxation?
- Do you overdo things such that you wear out completely by the end of the day or end of the week?
- Are there tasks you could relegate to others but don't?
- Are you able to let go of some goals in order to conserve energy (e.g., having a clean kitchen floor?)
- Could you trade a more intensive labor task for one involving less physical labor (e.g., you pay the bills and let someone else set the table)?
- Do you have things to do each day and week that interest you and give you enjoyment?

this affects our partnerships. Any problems between partners are likely to become more pronounced as stress increases. Thus, effects of polio/PPS and changes in functioning can make problems more apparent. An additional stress results from the differences in our expectations for how men versus women behave. For example, it is still unusual for a married woman to be the sole financial provider for her family. These societal views are unfortunate because they restrict free negotiations of roles and functions between couples. Partners need four main skills to successfully reach agreements on their relationship: (1) ability to express how they feel without blaming the other, and to listen to and validate the partner's feelings; (2) ability to set aside emotional expression to allow focused problem solving; (3) ability to negotiate until agreements are reached; and (4) willingness to make changes in their own behaviors. Negotiation is a fluid process; new information, feelings, or other changes require a return to the four skills listed here to reach a new agreement. Areas that may need discussion and negotiation vary from couple to couple, but there are some common areas. One is the balance of tasks between partners. Even couples without disabilities often have to negotiate the division of labor; however, as PPS symptoms increase, changes in duties may result so that old agreements no longer apply. It may be that the post-polio person takes on more of the less physical tasks, such as paying bills, making shopping lists, menu planning, and vacation arrangements. However, even as an agreement is reached, it is subject to change. We're not the only ones getting older; our partners are too. They may have changing abilities over time, and partners can become the one with the greater degree of disability, forcing a rebalancing of the relationship. The changes in your children's ages and stages of development will also require a rebalancing. As they increase their independence, leave home, pursue college and careers, bring prospective partners to Thanksgiving, have children of their own, and move away or move closer, the nature of their relationship with you will change. Some can provide financial, practical, or emotional assistance, and others will be less available. As always, the parents' relationship with their children will both reflect and alter the relationship between the couple.

Another area for negotiation is how assistance with personal care will be handled. Partners need to decide whether the more able-bodied partner will take on some of the care-giving tasks. As partners perform more intimate care-giving (for example, bathing the mate), a variety of feelings may arise. Some might feel closer to each other, the two of them tackling life together. Others may feel that as they do more care-giving, they become less of an equal partnership; the result may be that the nondisabled person's feelings of romance and sexual arousal for the partner with a disability seem to diminish. As one woman said to me, "I decided I could either be a wife or a nurse to my husband, but I couldn't be both." Feelings will vary from couple to couple; there is no one right feeling, decision, or way of being.

You and Your Children—Parenting with a Disability

Parenting is hard; parenting as a person with a disability is even harder. The first problem is that you probably don't have many (or even any) role models for how to be a parent with a disability. Obtaining general parenting support is an excellent idea because most of your concerns and struggles are common to all parents. However, you also will have concerns and questions specific to parenting with a disability.

Like other parents with disabilities, you've probably struggled with needing extra help, but you don't want to burden your child or have him or her do inappropriate tasks for you. Should you ask your three-year-old to pick up something you just dropped? Ask your five-year-old to go get the newspaper from the driveway, or ask your twelve-year-old to unload the groceries? How do you walk that fine line between teaching your children responsibility and helpfulness, courtesy and care, without crossing over into what professionals like to call "parentification"? This term means asking children to give up their childhoods to take on tasks vacated by parents. For example, I try to teach my children that in families we all help each other. But should I ask one of them to get something out of the dryer (at the other end of the house) for me because it's a long walk? What guidelines are there to help me decide this? One might ask several questions to decide what is appropriate. One is the age of the child. If my daughter is afraid to go down the hall and around the corner by herself at night because it's dark and the lights are off (a common fear at age six), it would not be good to force her. A second consideration is the child's freedom to say no. A third is whether the task has psychological or emotional overtones (e.g., a son giving a bath to his mother). These guidelines may seem clear on paper, but in practice, it's a hard row to hoe.

Your children are going to be exposed to others' attitudes, stereotypes, and assumptions about disability and about your fitness as a parent with a disability. We have to guide our children in developing their reactions to your disability, making room for any questions they may have (both those asked and those unasked). In addition, we have to help them manage their responses to other people's views, comments, and questions. How do people feel when they encounter a person with a serious disability? According to a recent Harris Poll (1995), the majority (92 percent) say they often or occasionally feel admiration, 74 percent feel pity, 58 percent feel awkward or embarrassed, 16 percent experience anger because persons with disabilities cause inconvenience, and nine percent feel resentment because persons with disabilities get special privileges.

How you respond to these feelings in others is what you are modeling to your children. At least five choices are available for how to respond. One is to rehearse your responses in advance by role-playing them with your family. A second choice is to ignore unwanted comments. This choice can convey discomfort, but if you've discussed it with your kids in advance ("We're going to ignore ignorant comments people make; we don't have to listen to that"), you can help them see it as an active choice. A third choice is to develop assertive responses, standing up to others, telling them how you feel, being honest. Although many of us probably do this with friends, admittedly it is harder to do with acquaintances, coworkers, or strangers. A fourth choice is to provide a simple explanation, which doesn't have to be medical ("I have symptoms of post-polio syndrome") but can describe the symptom ("I have some trouble with my hands"). This response can ease the situation and make it less likely that others will attribute your behavior to other things (for example, they might think you are not helping). Fifth, you can learn who accepts your disability and treats you as you'd like and spend more time with them, and less with those whose actions or comments are less helpful to you. Overall, it is healthier for you to spend time with people who accept and support you.

The task of parenting is complicated by lack of physical accessibility in many arenas. One such place is our children's schools, which are set up to be accessible to students with disabilities, not their parents with disabilities. For example, at my children's elementary school the day-care center has a ramp into the children's playroom, but not to the front desk where parents are to sign their children in and out. Recreation areas are another problem, as most parks and play centers (e.g., miniature golf, bowling, video arcades, skating rinks) are inaccessible. Many parents with disabilities develop alternate arenas for time with their children or have them go with other kids and their parents. Sometimes, the kids can't do some activities until they can do them more independently. But it's not so terrible if your child doesn't go ice-skating. So often we assume a deficit model; we focus on what they cannot do and assume that children of parents with disabilities are missing out. However, many children of able-bodied parents don't get to go ice-skating either. Disability becomes a convenient rack on which to hang our hats of guilt. Furthermore, children *gain* something from having a parent with a disability. Many reports indicate that such children are more tolerant of diversity and have greater empathy for others.

ROMANCE AND SEXUALITY

We as survivors have the same needs as others regarding sexual expression and the desire to lead a full life as people, partners, and parents. This section contains discussions on dating and romance, sexuality, pregnancy and childbirth, and lastly on aging.

Dating and Romance

For those without intimate romantic partners, disability may complicate the search for a mate. You may have a fear of rejection based on your very real experiences with negative responses to your disability, but in general, adults are kinder than children about disabilities. Are your fears based on old responses? You do need a skill that most people don't need, which is how to "contain" the disability, i.e., how to get people to see you as a person, not a disability, and how to help people understand that the disability affects only a small portion of what you can do. You need to know how to *present* the disability to others, to decrease their anxiety, and to come across as someone with a positive self-image. You also need to know how to answer questions about your disability and to fit the depth of the explanation to the situation and level of intimacy. Your comfort level with your disability will set the tone much more than does the extent of your disability. Yes, there are people out there who are not interested in a romantic relationship with someone with a visible disability. You know what the response is to that: for your well-being, you cannot be in a close relationship with someone who cannot accept your disability, but then you knew that already.

Sexuality

Sexuality is not one thing, but a series of interactive factors. Sexual desire and sexual functioning are not the same thing; they are two interrelated but separate components of sexuality. Each of these may be affected by polio/PPS. Many variables affect sexuality in persons with PPS, including the nature of the disability itself: severity, how the body is affected, age at onset of polio, current age and combined effects of aging and PPS. A second factor is the nature of the relationship with a partner, whether the partner also has a disability and the partner's attitudes toward disability and sexuality. A third factor affecting sexuality has to do with how one sees oneself. Do you have a positive body image overall? How are your skills in social interactions, romance, and sex? Many persons with disabilities are seen as asexual. How were you raised to see yourself? Do you see yourself as a sexual person? Remember, sex isn't just something one *does*; a sexual person is something one *is*. Increasing sexual interest and pleasure may not be so much a matter of changing sexual behaviors as it is making other changes, notably increasing physical comfort, decreasing pain and fatigue. If pain, fatigue, and weakness are the primary symptoms of PPS, then sexuality is directly affected by PPS. Therefore the reduction of its symptoms can enhance sexual interest and functioning. Strength or weakness of limbs may affect choice of positions. Some medications (e.g., for spasms) or some antidepressants can affect sexual desire and functioning. Probably one of the biggest factors is fatigue. Finding times in the day or week when energy levels are more optimum is not always easy. Sexual innovation is generally useful, such as finding positions that promote relaxation and don't tax muscles, or widening the array of pleasurable activities.

Sexual encounters may become less spontaneous and more planned. Time of day can be important for some people, taking into consideration needs such as warming up muscles, ensuring reasonable levels of energy and avoiding fatigue, or timing in relation to when medications are taken.

How old you were when you had polio probably affected how you think of yourself, your body, and your sexuality. If the onset was relatively late (post-adolescence), you already had a prior history of sexuality before the onset of polio. For those who had polio at a younger age, your sense of sexual self-identity and development included the polio. But it isn't only your own self-image that was affected by the polio. The ways others viewed you and treated you were also affected by your disability. Too often persons with disabilities are treated as asexual beings. Role models of persons with disabilities active in all spheres of life, including sexuality, are sorely lacking. Perhaps your doctors treated you as a body part—an affected leg, for example, that only incidentally happened to have been attached to *you*. You may have thought of yourself this way; many of us talk about our *good* parts (e.g., the good leg) and bad parts (e.g., the bad leg), thinking of ourselves as split into two. Which part contains our sexual selves?

Although the findings from studies are not consistent, a U.S. government report places the risk of sexual abuse for people with disabilities at 1.7 times the rate of those without disabilities. It is likely that sexual abuse of children with disabilities is even more under-reported than for nondisabled children. People with disabilities face additional barriers (e.g., access to transportation) that impede reporting. We can only speculate about the reasons for any increased rate of abuse of children with disabilities: increased physical dependence, reduced independence, engendering negative feelings in the adults, increased physical vulnerability, and reduced believability when reporting abuse. Incidence of acquaintance or "date rape" may also be increased; lack of social opportunities can make people with disabilities feel beholden to anyone who seems to take a sexual interest in them or are more willing to "settle" for what they can get. Fewer dating opportunities may mean that the person with a disability has less chance to practice skills in self-assertion and protection or is less able to recognize early signs of potential danger. Any and all of these reasons could account for increased vulnerability to abuse for people with disabilities. The presence of a history of such abuse does not necessarily mean that you will experience sexual or intimacy difficulties later in life, but does make them more probable. Addressing such difficulties should include the assistance of a trained professional.

Perhaps sexuality was missing as a topic in your development. You may have experienced a lack of opportunities for sexual exploration. Being a teenager with a disability may have inhibited social interactions and reduced dating and romantic or intimate connections. Thus, you may have been a "late bloomer." Because persons with disabilities are often ostracized as children and adolescents, they have fewer opportunities for social interactions, less practice in social skills, and less feedback on their social functioning. However, early onset of a disability does not mean that the person has more problems or is less *adjusted.* In fact, a national survey of parents with disabilities suggests that those with earlier onset had integrated the disability more into their self-concept. Self-concept in turn affects sexuality. If that self-concept is negatively affected by disability, then sexuality will be too.

It is easy, but often erroneous, to ascribe any sexual difficulties to polio/PPS. As we age, we may too readily accept that sexuality will decrease, and be too resigned and accepting of decreased sexual interest or pleasure. We should not presume that all negative effects on our bodies are caused by polio. Any chronic pain or discomfort should be checked out by a medical professional. Changes in desire or functioning should also be investigated. While these may be caused by increased fatigue or pain related to PPS, other causes must be ruled out. For example, I went for more than six months attributing my considerably lessened energy level to worsening of PPS symptoms, when it turned out I had a thyroid problem!

Sex can be a barometer signaling difficulties in other areas. Sexuality can mirror general psychological and emotional functioning, the relationship with one's partner, and one's own physical health. Relationship conflicts, family stresses, poor health, depression, anxiety, work or financial problems—any of these can impact sexuality. Therefore, sexuality must be addressed in the context of the whole person. Oftentimes remedies for sexual difficulties require little to no outside intervention. However, in some instances it is helpful to consult a professional. To be of help to you, that professional needs to possess certain skills. These skills might be thought of as falling into one of four levels. At the first level is the ability to give *permission*. This ability involves helping you feel okay about being sexual, making it a priority, being able to initiate and respond sexually. One of the most important aspects in alleviating any sexual difficulties is to help the person feel *normal*. Most people think their sexual problems are unique, weird, abnormal, deviant. Thus, talking with others is a good way to feel more *normal*. For persons with polio, talking with other persons with polio can be enormously reassuring. Talking with persons with other disabilities also can be quite helpful. As discussed in an earlier chapter, persons with disabilities share much in common, and sexual concerns constitute one area in which we can help each other. If a professional is consulted for this level of intervention, no special training is necessary for a professional to give this kind of assistance.

The next level of assistance is *general information*; this assistance also can be provided by most professionals, including information about the effects of a medication on sexual functioning, dispelling myths, or providing factual information. However, *specific suggestions* tailored to your particular needs may require someone with more training, either about disability or about sexuality (preferably both). Too often professionals with training in one of these areas lack training in the other, making holistic treatment more difficult to obtain. To make specific suggestions requires that someone get to know more about you and your sexual history, and about your specific disability and its manifestations. For example, advice about what to do with a Foley catheter could only come from a professional trained in disability issues. (Dr. Halstead suggests that you can tape it out of the way or remove it temporarily and reduce liquid intake prior.) For assistance at this level, professionals should have some specific training and experience in sex counseling.

The final level of assistance may involve more *focused treatment* about issues connected to sexuality (e.g., marital therapy, treatment for the aftermath of sexual abuse). Professionals providing this type of care should be well-trained and experienced in this type of work. Ideally, they should be well-versed in both sexuality and disability, even if not specifically in polio/PPS. This hierarchy of assistance needs is not meant to imply that those with more in-depth needs are hopeless, more damaged or abnormal. Rather, it is intended as a way to help readers understand different types of assistance that are available and how to evaluate the level of training of any professional consulted.

Of course, all the factors in sexuality for persons without disabilities still apply to persons with polio/PPS, including issues such as AIDS and safer sexual practices, sexual attitudes, sexual preferences, history of sexual and/or physical abuse, and substance use or abuse. Polio/PPS cannot be the scapegoat for all problems, and other issues should not be overshadowed by the fact of disability. We want to be treated as whole people, so we must think of ourselves this way as well.

Pregnancy and Childbirth

Because of the general age of the group of persons who had polio (over 40), probably most of us who were going to "commit parenthood" have already done so. But for those still deciding, there are some disability issues to consider. Polio generally does not affect fertility. Your age is one factor to weigh in deciding whether and when to get pregnant. All women do better (i.e., recover faster and have fewer complications) when they have babies in their twenties compared to their thirties. This fact is especially important for many women with disabilities. The effects of aging (even in your thirties), polio/PPS, and pregnancy can combine to produce more symptoms in pregnancy. The question is not so much how does the disability affect the pregnancy (in general, polio is not a problem), but rather how does the pregnancy affect the disability. Many women report increased fatigue beyond that expected from pregnancy, which continues through the three trimesters. There may be increases in muscle weakness and in pain. With the additional weight in the third trimester, mobility may be impaired. None of this is meant to discourage pregnancy, but to help women plan for it more realistically. Nonetheless, a positive approach to pregnancy and parenting is recommended.

Once pregnant, remember that you know your body best, so be actively involved in all decisions. You are first and foremost a pregnant woman, not a disabled woman, and should be treated as such. However, you are the expert on your disability, and you are the best one to know if the pregnancy is affecting your disability. You may need to seek consultation from outside the ob/gyn group. In any case a team approach is recommended. Possible other participants in your pregnancy include your partner/coach, your primary birth/delivery doctor or nurse midwife, your primary physician for disability, and the anesthesiologist.

Labor and delivery can be affected by several aspects of polio, such as weakened stomach muscles, scoliosis, or pelvic deformity. These may make preplanned cesarean birth preferable. Careful evaluation of the pros and cons of vaginal versus cesarean births should be undertaken. Recovery from a cesarean birth is generally longer than from vaginal deliveries, but labor may overwork muscles and leave the mother with increased pain, weakness, and even temporary paralysis during post-delivery recovery. Pain medication and anesthesia also need careful analysis. Results of one study of pregnancy and childbirth in mothers with disabilities suggest that epidurals can cause temporary paralysis in polio-affected limbs.

Aging

It used to be that I could go to a new orthopedist and the doctor would look at my ankle and say, "I see you had a triple arthrodesis [ankle fusion]." Today, an M.D. is likely to look at the scar and ask how I got it, and I'm likely to be his or her first polio patient. Thus, one effect of aging is that our numbers are dwindling, and the number of professionals with experience in polio is likewise diminishing. This fact makes me feel old. Getting older combines with the effects of polio/PPS. Although many people slow with age, this process is more rapid or pronounced for us. The onset of PPS coupled with effects of aging is like acquiring a second disability, or the first one all over again. The meaning of aging for us is different than for others because it reawakens old feelings associated with the onset of our polio. We have to integrate our increasing disability into a self-concept that was also being assaulted by the aging process.

Persons who are older and have disabilities fall into two camps: those with disabilities who are aging (like us) and those who become older and experience a disability. The experiences of these two groups are not equivalent. Those of us with disabilities acquired early in life are not entering our later years from a level playing field. We come with some disadvantages; those with disabilities generally have less education, more unemployment, lower income, and higher levels of poverty. Additionally, our disabilities may have increased our need for support from family or service agencies, higher medical costs, and financial costs associated with modifying the environment to increase its accessibility and with assistive devices. Further, relatively minor physical deterioration may be more pronounced for us when combined with our PPS symptoms. Often we experience a decrease in functioning earlier than others do. However, we also come with some strengths; we have been members of a disadvantaged group of lower status (persons with disabilities) and hence have learned ways of coping prior to entering a second group of lower status (the elderly). We've developed ways to cope with functional losses. Further, we've gained wisdom through experience. We've learned that we have to prioritize *everything*, give up on some items further down the list of priorities, and make compromises.

We must be especially mindful of our increased physical vulnerability. Women in particular should be taking extra calcium to offset osteoporosis. It is a good idea to install aids before they are needed, such as grab bars around a shower/tub, handles around the toilet, ramps to the front step, or an extra handrail on stairs. Find ways now to ease your load. For example, put a phonebook, pen, and notepad next to each phone in the house to avoid walking to get supplies.

Disability is not an inevitable experience of aging, and most older people do not have disabilities. More than 60 percent of older people report that their health is good or excellent, although some might take their age into consideration in making this evaluation ("I'm in pretty good shape considering my years"). Most (about 80 percent) can live independently and care for themselves, even with chronic health problems. Nonetheless, aging usually means deterioration of some functions (usually hearing and vision), more susceptibility to injury, and quicker onset of fatigue. All of these problems may be more noticeable for us, and unlike the gradual onset for our peers, we may experience sudden decreases of functioning. Once again, we are faced with an unpredictable course of our disabilities, one requiring continual readjustments.

One hallmark of older age is retirement. Retirement is often the result, rather than the cause, of poor health. Many of us may retire at earlier ages than we might have without our disabilities or take advantage of a job change to leave the workforce. Retirement in the late fifties, say, puts us out of synch with our peers, who may continue working for at least another decade. Before retiring, employees should take advantage of any group insurance plans offered. For example, persons with polio/PPS may be denied long-term care insurance if they try to buy it individually, but the plan offered at work may prohibit exclusion of any employees. For those with PPS, retirement can free up time and energy and allow a more evenly paced lifestyle without overfatigue. But with retirement comes a change in roles in the family; again, we need a fluid definition of roles and functions within the family.

Another frequent occurrence with age is widowhood, the single most disruptive and deleterious event affecting older persons. It is associated with increased illness and death in the surviving spouse. For those with disabilities it brings additional stresses. Any negative changes to income may be more pronounced for persons with disabilities because of increased need for aid (e.g., shopping), accessibility (e.g., installing grab bars), or convenience (e.g., buying prepared meals). The loss of daily practical and emotional support and of interdependence makes us more vulnerable to institutionalization. Because losing a spouse is so emotionally overwhelming, it is difficult to cope with the loss and make new practical plans simultaneously. For example, the spouse may have provided tangible support (e.g., aiding you in and out of the bathtub, driving, preparing meals, help with shopping and laundry), which will have to be found elsewhere. It is wise to set up backup plans, a support system, and alternate means of aid before they are needed. Even if you never use them, just knowing the options can alleviate anxiety and be immediately useful at a time of loss.

As we age, we lose other significant persons to illness and death, and these losses can take an emotional toll. Our family (parents, siblings, spouses, children) are also aging and may become less able to provide support. Hospitalization of loved ones or of oneself can re-evoke earlier hospital traumas connected with polio onset or surgeries.

Although there are many potential negatives associated with aging, there are also many positives. One is that our disabilities become more "normal" among our peers. As they age some begin to acquire disabilities, so that having a disability is less rare. We go from being a member of a minority group to just one of the gang. Older age can be a time for evaluation and reflection, increased wisdom and maturity, freedom from caring so much about what others think, new interests, and fewer demands. To enjoy these, it is important that we maintain good health practices, continue to get exercise, and be active. Too often the view of older age as a time of inevitably declining health leads people (including professionals) to minimize the benefits of rehabilitation. Since rehabilitation usually means restoring function and increasing independence, these may not be seen as realistic goals for older persons. Further, our health-care system is more oriented toward treatment of acute, short-term problems, and is less proficient in providing ongoing care, while persons with polio/PPS have a chronic condition. These views of older persons with disabilities unnecessarily limit our options. We should not give in too readily to these notions, but strive to remain active and involved.

As we age, money helps enormously. People generally need time (to do the task) or money (to hire someone else to do the task). Whoever says you can't throw money at a problem doesn't have a disability. Disability is a problem that money can ameliorate tremendously: Wheelchair breaks too often? Buy a new one. Fatigue interfering with family life? Hire a cook. Can't drive? Hire a driver. Money does wonders. Even without lots of money, little things can make a difference. Sometimes the problem is in not knowing how valuable a change, addition, or assistive device will be until one tries it. For example, we raised our living room so it was no longer sunken by one step. Only then did I realize how much I had avoided the living room. That one step made all the difference. You have to look for the steps in your life, real and metaphorical, and ramp them.

9

Journeying Together: Post-Polio Support Groups

NANCY BALDWIN CARTER
RUTH WILDER BELL

Interest in post-polio support groups (PPSGs) increased dramatically in the United States during the 1980s. This interest was in large part caused by the influence of Gini Laurie, longtime publisher of *Polio Gazette* and champion of polio survivors around the world. Laurie laid the foundation of the polio support group movement when she organized a conference in Chicago in October 1981. Among those who attended were physicians and other health-care providers concerned about the long-term neglect of polio survivors. More importantly, the conference brought together hundreds of individuals who had begun experiencing the late effects of polio. For the first time, it gave these people an opportunity to meet together, share experiences, and discuss the implications of their troubling symptoms.

Out of the exchanges at this conference came the idea of polio survivors uniting in common cause to organize and meet in support groups wherever there was a need. Without any formal structure or national organization to fund or financially promote this effort, a nationwide *grass-roots* phenomenon began to occur. Almost overnight, support groups started springing up in cities and towns all across the country. Today, there are approximately 300 PPSGs in 45 states and many more in other countries. Although each group is unique, PPSGs share many common concerns and characteristics.

PURPOSE

Individuals are drawn to groups when they believe that being with others improves the chances of meeting their personal needs and achieving goals with the group that cannot be accomplished alone. Polio survivors have significant reasons for joining with one another. Their lives are changing in puzzling and sometimes frightening ways. These changes may be accompanied by feelings of isolation, anxiety and/or depression. Family and friends, to whom they normally turn for comfort, may not understand these new symptoms and at times urge individuals in directions their bodies can no longer go. Survivors need the emotional support of others in the same situation; they need information about what is happening to their bodies; and they need help in finding resources. Many of these needs can be met in PPSGs.

Support groups also meet the needs of friends and family members. The late effects of polio affect more people than the polio survivor alone. Those who care about someone who has lived through the polio experience have their own questions and worries. Participation in a support group offers family and friends, as well as the polio survivor, opportunities to voice concerns and fears and to gain information and practical assistance in improving their quality of life.

GETTING STARTED: FINDING POLIO SURVIVORS AND THOSE WHO CARE ABOUT THEM

Knowledge of the workings of the local community aids in finding polio survivors. Announcements in local papers and on local radio stations, messages on a cable TV company's community bulletin board, and messages on post-polio web sites are among the possibilities. Brochures can be left at health-care locations frequented by polio survivors. Even more effective than announcements in local papers and on television are newspaper and television human interest features focusing on people living with post-polio. Support groups typically report an increase in calls requesting information together with an increase in attendance following such publicity.

One support group reported success in placing posters throughout a region in all the grocery stores in a large chain. Others have reported using the powerful network of polio survivors who were hospitalized together and have kept in contact over the years as a means of building membership in a support group.

Finding a Meeting Place

Limited funding is a given for most support groups. Thus, finding a meeting place that is free, or rents for very little money, is an important goal. Some hospitals and other health-care institutions are willing to provide backing for support groups by offering meeting space. Public libraries and churches are other possibilities, as are senior centers. The Easter Seal Society and the March of Dimes may have meeting rooms available together with independent living centers. Corporations with a community outreach focus may be willing to donate a room. Other issues to consider in choosing a location relate to the accessibility of the facility, the availability of accessible restrooms, and the presence of adequate handicapped parking.

Meeting Time and Frequency of Meetings

While it is important to choose a time convenient for the greatest number of people, experienced support group leaders have found that the choice of a particular time is less important than the consistency of both time and location. Typically, PPSGs are scheduled once a month. People will develop the habit of returning to worthwhile meetings held at the same hour, day, and place each month.

LEADERSHIP

By definition a support group is a collection of people with common experiences who draw strength from others with similar backgrounds and come together for a common purpose. Thus, it is unusual for support groups to be assigned a professional leader. However, many professionals, such as psychologists, social workers, nurses, or physicians, are polio survivors and may be designated the group leader. The leader has primary responsibility for keeping a meeting running and attending to the emotional climate of that meeting. However, this role is but one aspect of the leadership necessary for a successful support group. As it is unwieldy for all the members to make ongoing decisions about group life, it is useful to have a smaller group of people who serve as a planning or oversight committee. This committee is entrusted with a variety of responsibilities from ongoing program planning to making arrangements for a meeting place and publicity. Sharing these responsibilities encourages broader participation, helps develop a sense of commitment among a greater number of people, and protects the group from domination by one person.

THE MEETING

PPSGs have two major functions: (1) to provide emotional support for those caught in the often confusing and frustrating changes of an unfamiliar physical condition and (2) to provide an opportunity for members to gain insight and make life changes as they learn from one another and the group's educational experiences.

Meeting Emotional Needs

In a support group, the emotional needs of members are increasingly met as closeness develops and the members become more like a community. Becoming involved means a willingness to be identified with that group and to risk connection with others with the same affiliation. Thus, closeness becomes a central goal of support groups as they evolve through a series of stages, stages characteristic of the development of all groups. Five stages of group life were identified in the 1960s by the Boston University School of Social Work. Knowing about these stages is helpful in guiding a support group to grow and mature. These five stages are defined as (1) pre-affiliation, (2) power and control, (3) intimacy, (4) differentiation, and (5) separation. Each stage is described below.

Pre-affiliation

This stage is characterized by *approach-avoidance* behavior, that is, individuals at one moment seem involved and ready to make a commitment to the group and at the next moment, they withdraw and may not seem interested at all. Attendance may be sporadic, reflective of the general ambivalence regarding identification with other members of the group or with the goals or activities of the group. (Approach-avoidance behavior is especially characteristic of polio survivors who have *passed* as normal for most of their lives.) The role of the leader during this phase is to allow and support this cautious *arms-length* exploration while at the same time patiently inviting trust and involvement.

Power and Control

During this stage, members who have resolved their ambivalence about involvement in the group begin to make arrangements to handle some of its work. The designated leader is seen as the one holding the power and is still held responsible by the members for the group's success. Competition among individuals for attention from the leader is characteristic of member behavior. An effective leader, however, does not respond to the competition for attention and treats all members as equals, encouraging them to take increasing responsibility for the success of the organization's efforts. As this stage closes, members have made a significant investment in the group and have accepted some responsibility for its success and survival.

Intimacy

Group cohesion and a sense of belonging flourish during this stage. The group is now seen as a safe place in which feelings can be expressed and new experiences tried. The group looks less and less to the leader as a source of gratification or for solutions to problems. Members increasingly accept and share responsibility for group functioning and are able to carry out its various tasks and objectives.

Differentiation

During this stage, the growth of closeness and the level of intimacy that became apparent during the preceding stage continue. There is increasing recognition and acceptance of individual needs. A unique situation has been created that allows for group cohesion with the group's own personality and expectations of members, while the integrity of individual members is fully respected. The leader is needed less and less and the group increasingly runs itself.

Separation

Separation occurs when the group has met its purpose and the members are ready to move on, taking with them what they have learned from the experience. As members prepare to leave the group, they may revert to old behaviors, looking once again to the leader for direction. An appropriate role for the leader is to *let go*, encouraging members to review both the group's accomplishments and what they as individuals have learned from participating. Particularly useful is a discussion of how experiences in the group can be transferred to new situations.

Guiding a support group through these stages and mobilizing the strengths that come with the cohesion and closeness of the later stages are not easy matters. A characteristic of support groups that makes this task more difficult is that several things may happen at the same time. A core of members may continue to attend regularly and represent the *culture bearers*. A second pool of people may cycle in and out, perhaps not having resolved their initial ambivalence about attending, or perhaps returning each time their post-polio symptoms get worse. This second group of people needs to be *caught up* or reoriented each time its members attend. To add to the challenge at any meeting, there may be those who are attending for the first time and aren't sure what the group is all about and whether they even want to participate!

The core members, those who cycle in and out, and the newcomers are in different places emotionally. It is the leader's task to respect their needs to be close or not close, and to set the stage for an environment in which individual differences are respected and individual needs can be met. Below are a few suggestions to help create such an environment:

- Have someone available to greet newcomers, provide name tags and introductions, and give an orientation to the group.
- Plan for social time before and after the program.
- Remind the group at each meeting that what is discussed during the program is confidential. (This is often a concern for those who believe their job security is affected by their physical abilities.)
- Encourage core members to discuss what it was like for them when they first began attending. Hopefully, this will make it easier to begin talking and sharing for those who are not ready for the same level of intimacy as the others.
- Watch new members, or those who attend sporadically, for signs of discomfort if the discussion involves significant sharing. At the end of the meeting, the leader might speak privately to these persons, letting them know that they will not be pressured to do or say anything that makes them uncomfortable.
- Respect the right of members to attend at intervals, depending on their need and readiness for the group. The leader can express interest in these individuals by making arrangements for another member to call periodically just to say, "Hello." Delegating to another member conveys the notion that members share responsibility for the group. It is not the leader's job alone.
- Begin each meeting with a *check-in*. This is a time when members catch up with each other since the last meeting. Because sharing is voluntary, it protects those who are not ready to participate but also communicates that the meeting is a safe place for members to share with each other, should they desire to do so.
- As beneficial as support groups are, some individuals have a need more appropriately met by professional counseling.
- A leader and members can do many other things to provide an environment in which needs can be met. The leader might invite the entire group to participate in a discussion of ways the members can meet the needs of those who are at different levels of involvement with the group. Such a discussion communicates a sense of shared responsibility for the life of the

group. Time devoted to nurturing the group as a whole, as well as the individuals in the group, is time well spent.

Meeting Educational and Social Needs

While a program committee is often given the responsibility for program planning and implementation, support groups find it useful to occasionally spend part or all of a meeting brainstorming new program ideas and group goals. Ideas for the use of meeting time and a rationale for continuing are then limited only by the creativity of the group. When outside speakers are needed, there are numerous options in every community. Many health-care professionals are willing to share their expertise. Physicians, psychologists, family therapists, social workers, nutritionists, occupational therapists, physical therapists, acupuncturists, massage therapists, and exercise physiologists, among others, have knowledge and skills to help polio survivors understand their unique situation better and make appropriate lifestyle choices. Certified public accountants, disability lawyers, architects familiar with accessibility issues, and specialists in retirement and in the use of leisure time are others in the community who may be helpful. Community colleges and universities often have a speakers' bureau. Representatives from disability-related organizations (e.g., the Easter Seal Society, Paralyzed Veterans of America, Centers for Independent Living) might be invited to present an overview of the services of the organization or the organization's views on a particular topic relevant to managing post-polio problems.

When an outside presenter has been invited to meet with the group, it is important to provide time for interaction of the members with the speaker as well as among one another. Videos from regional or national post-polio conferences, followed by discussion are helpful. Field trips to points of interest in the community, such as accessible recreational facilities, provide a different pace. Social activities, picnics, potluck suppers and lunch together contribute variety.

Dealing with Support Group Burn Out

Sometimes, a topical discussion *without* an outside speaker might be the program for the month. Always having an *outsider* for each meeting may be a way of avoiding difficult issues the group needs to discuss on its own: issues such as attendance, membership dues, finances, leader *burn-out*, group relevance, future goals, etc. There are times when discussing difficult issues openly and honestly will create a healthy *crisis*, which paradoxically may generate fresh enthusiasm and energy in the life of the group. Finally, some PPSGs have made connections with other disease-specific disability groups, such as multiple sclerosis and stroke.

While these diseases and others may be very different from polio, many of the disability issues and support group concerns are similar. Sharing program ideas, experiences with community resources, and strategies for enhancing support group growth and effectiveness can be beneficial for everyone.

SUMMARY

As polio survivors and those who care about them wrestle with the chaos caused by new disability, support groups help in bringing lives back into focus. Learning about post-polio syndrome within the supportive community of others making the same journey provides understanding, hope, and an awareness of the many options available to improve the quality of life. Adjusting to change is made easier as people are nourished by the sense of togetherness that is available nowhere else. Some come to the group, receive what they need, and leave to carry on life, never to return. Others leave and return only when symptoms flare. Still others who cherish the ongoing relationship with group members continue to attend even after their initial needs have been met. As some members depart, the group is replenished by newcomers. They are beginning their search for understanding and acceptance of new losses knowing what those who have come before them have known: some things are done more easily in a group of people with similar experiences than done alone. The cycle continues.

Portions of this chapter were previously published in the Polio Network News.

—10—
Vocational Strategies

BEVERLY NEWAY
LIINA PAASUKE
NANCY E. BOGG

Throughout one's work life, questions arise regarding success. Success can be measured from a financial perspective, but more often it also involves the issue of meeting one's needs through meaningful activities. With the changing needs in the job market, you may be facing adjustments in your current work. When this is compounded with post-polio health concerns, you may want to reevaluate your long-term vocational and avocational goals.

Disabilities from post-polio may affect personal and professional functions alike. The process of understanding the possibilities and re-establishing goals may seem overwhelming. *It is critical to remember that it is a process, not a quick fix.* The amount of time needed to complete this process varies greatly from person to person.

Working through the psychological aspects of change is vital. Your energy will be needed to gather information and solve problems. Your family, counseling services, and support groups can help you cope with changes and identify strategies for regaining control. To examine your work capacity and the requirements of various jobs, a vocational rehabilitation counselor (VR counselor) can help to explore options fully and craft a plan that will work for you in the workplace or in the classroom.

The measure of success for this process is not simply obtaining or preserving a job. Success is fully achieved when realistic goals are set and the challenges they represent are met. It may not be feasible for some to retain employment, so it is vital to remember that personal worth is not contingent on being employed. *What is important is to be engaged in something that has meaning for you.* Volunteers and mentors of all types are sorely needed; this work can be combined with your own interests or hobbies. Vocational counseling can help you pull together the best package possible and explore personal goals and interests.

VOCATIONAL REHABILITATION COUNSELING SERVICES

A VR counselor can be the key in assessing and coordinating needs. The professional training of most VR counselors includes a Bachelor's degree and a Master's degree in rehabilitation counseling, guidance counseling, or another related field. The VR counselor should have one or more national certifications as a certified rehabilitation counselor or certified disability management specialist.

VR counselors work for state vocational rehabilitation agencies, private rehabilitation agencies, medical centers, centers for independent living, or insurance companies. Services are available at no charge through the state agencies and the centers for independent living. If a person is receiving long-term disability benefits, the insurer may pay for these services, sometimes through an employee assistance program. Vocational counselors, without specialized rehabilitation knowledge, are also available through state employment security commissions, and through college counseling and placement offices at no charge.

Public programs provide a wide range of services to help people with disabilities obtain or return to employment. If one is considered eligible for services by meeting the specific criteria established, the services and resources are free. The disadvantages of these resources are that personnel have limited knowledge about such concerns as accommodation of needs, there is often a waiting list for eligibility determination, and there tends to be a focus on short-term services. These services include: (1) vocational evaluation, (2) specific vocational training, and (3) employment placement rather than long-term accommodation of needs and follow-up.

Private individuals who specialize in vocational counseling can be located through the yellow pages of the telephone book. Although these counselors may not have a rehabilitation background, they may be excellent resources for personal assessment and employment information.

The private VR counselor is likely to be more responsive than the publicly-funded professional. Most often, the private rehabilitation professional has worked with insurance-related, return-to-work issues as a member of a team with a large employer, as a counselor for a specific vocational rehabilitation company, or as an individual consultant. The downside to this resource, however, is payment arrangements. It may require working directly with health-care providers so that referrals can be made by a treating physician and authorized through the insurance policy. Once the process has started, additional funding options can be recommended by the vocational rehabilitation professional for needs such as equipment modifications and job accommodations.

The services provided by the VR counselor are:

- Assessment of individual educational and vocational abilities which include intelligence, work-related aptitudes, vocational interests, academics, and transferable skills.
- Provision of counseling services which include prevocational, individual, group, and job-seeking skills to assist individuals with vocational adjustment and community reintegration goals.
- Provision of work skills training which may include simulated work activities to prepare individuals for competitive employment opportunities.
- Facilitation of specialized services, including employer or school consultations, school or work site evaluation and accommodations, job analysis, and selective placement options to assist individuals in returning to employment or school.
- Education of prospective employers or school officials concerning the vocational and educational implications of various disabilities to assure success. This includes providing information on accessibility, accommodation, and disability-related legislation affecting employment or education and working with people with disabilities.
- Following up with employer or education services to assist people with disabilities in maintaining employment or education placement.

To perform these services, the VR counselor must understand the needs of the employer, the demands of the job, and the capabilities of the client. The task of the VR counselor is to assist individuals in meeting their goals and bridge the gap between disability and work. The VR counselor may be particularly helpful if an employer is resistant to providing accommodations. This resistance is often due to a lack of information and awareness about the assistance available to make the accommodations, the specific physical limitations of post-polio, and the requirements of the Americans with Disabilities Act (ADA). The VR counselor can provide education that helps ensure that employment is beneficial to both the client and the employer.

THE JOB ACCOMMODATION PROCESS

A comprehensive job accommodation process includes five phases: job analysis, functional capacity evaluation, job market, job search, and reasonable accommodations.

The Job Analysis

A systematic study of both the work tasks and the physical demands (ergonomic aspects) of the workplace must be reviewed. This review of the job tasks considers *how* and *when* they are accomplished and the expected outcomes. The VR counselor should examine job descriptions, tasks of the job, educational requirements, physical and mental demands of the environment, and employment outlook. The ergonomic job analysis is performed at the worksite by a qualified physical therapist (or occupational therapist if upper extremities are exclusively involved). The therapist measures the physical demands of the job and makes recommendations concerning ways to make the job more appropriate and ergonomically safer. When combined with the functional capacity information described below, the information from an ergonomic job analysis provides the basis for development and implementation of a successful work plan. Appropriate job tasks or workplace accommodations can then be recommended.

The Functional Capacity Evaluation

An evaluation of functional capacity requires an honest and accurate assessment of your abilities as they relate to specific job tasks. The evaluation is completed at a rehabilitation center, usually by an occupational therapist. Typically, this testing is not a covered benefit under insurance plans. The evaluation may include assessing your capacity for handling manual materials (lifting), aerobic capacity (cardio-respiratory fitness), posture and mobility tolerance (walking, sitting, bending, stooping, climbing, twisting), and anthropometric measurements (measurements of your body, size, weight and proportions). This evaluation involves measurement of actual work ability during simulated work tasks and computerized measurement of the force exerted isometrically during lifting tasks. The results of the evaluation are reviewed with you and the coordinating VR counselor. Each recommendation should be made on an individual basis. The recommendations might suggest specific pacing of tasks, healthy work posture, reasonable accommodations, or work redesign for your safety and productivity on the job.

The functional capacity evaluation may indicate that the person is unable to return to his/her previous occupation. In that case, the VR counselor may suggest aptitude and interest testing to help develop alternative vocational plans. If, for example, a person could no longer physically perform nursing duties and the position could not be accommodated, one would look at other settings where a nursing background might be helpful, e.g., an insurance company. If the insurance company position requires additional clerical duties, the evaluation might assess that person's computer or word-processing skills and indicate additional training. Training may be required in a new setting and a VR counselor would be able to assist in securing that training.

The Job Market

When considering new lines of work, the VR counselor's knowledge of the job market and availability of jobs is critical. Once several alternatives can be identified, informational interviews can be invaluable. Finding out what people do on a daily basis and reviewing their likes and dislikes can provide a more realistic picture of a job than reading the description.

The newspaper classified ads are often the least helpful resource in seeking employment. However, they may help identify trends. The U.S. Department of Labor publishes *The Occupational Outlook Handbook* every few years, which identifies the future job outlook. Most jobs are found through personal contacts and networking within your field of interest. The state department of employment offers job lists. Often, however, making cold calls can reap high rewards if they are done systematically.

The Job Search

Job-seeking skills are important and can be learned through coaching by the VR counselor, through many types of publications or job clubs that are available through the state departments of employment, or through publications. Job seeking skills include identifying and following up on job leads, resume writing, application completion, and interviewing skills. These skills are not unique to persons with disabilities. Many books are available on these topics at local libraries and bookstores. One helpful workbook is the *Job Seekers' Guide to Employment*. This book reviews (1) how to get the job you want, (2) selling yourself, (3) locating job leads, (4) feeling okay about yourself during your job search, (5) good telephone techniques, (6) interviewing skills, and (7) getting the job you want.

As a job applicant, you must be prepared to complete a variety of applications. The applications must be completed neatly and accurately with no blanks. Job skills need to be described in specific terms, both on the application and in the interview. For example, rather than stating "office work," you should be more descriptive, i.e., describe computer systems and programs used, keyboard speed, etc. Legally, an employer may ask only one question, "Do you have any condition or disability that would interfere with your ability to perform the tasks of this job?" If your disability would affect the performance of the job or is obvious to the eye, it should be briefly described, avoiding the use of medical terminology. This advice holds true for the application, the resume, and the interview. For example, rather than saying, "I have post-polio," it would be better to say, "I walk slowly and have difficulty picking up small objects," or, "I use a wheelchair to get around, but this would not interfere with my ability to do the job." Thus, the focus should be on your ability to do the job, rather than on the disability as a limitation.

It is usually better to discuss disability issues at an appropriate time in the interview, not on the application or resume. However, if there is a question on the application about this issue, you should answer the question with a request to discuss it at the time of the interview. All communication between you and the potential employer should focus on your skills and abilities, not on disability issues.

The resume is typically the first contact with employers. As such, it needs to be well organized, concise, and easy to read. Different resumes may be required to emphasize different skills. Again, there is no legal requirement for the disability to be addressed on the resume. However, if you have a visible disability, you may wish to avoid "surprising" the interviewer. Your disability could be stated in indirect ways, i.e., "Post-Polio support group member," or, "I qualify for the Affirmative Action Program under section 503 of the Rehabilitation Act," or, "Am active in wheelchair sports."

As a job applicant, you must be prepared to handle a wide range of interview styles and techniques. You must be practiced in your responses and prepared to initiate discussion of the disability as appropriate. It is also your responsibility to know what job accommodations you need. Role-playing and/or videotaping practice interviews with a VR counselor are effective tools to increase interviewing confidence. It is important to avoid yes/no answers and to be able to elaborate on your skills using specific examples whenever possible. The first five to ten minutes of the interview are critical since employers often make hiring decisions based on their first impressions. It is important to show enthusiasm and interest through voice tone and eye contact.

As the applicant, you need to be able to take the initiative in discussing the disability, especially if it is visible. You can address it directly, clear up any misconceptions, and speak to any concerns or questions the employer may have regarding the disability. Do not assume that the employer knows anything about the disability. Typical statements could include, "I have had this condition since childhood, and I've learned to do most things that other people can do."

Then you can give some examples. Another statement might be, "You may be wondering if I can be dependable; I have my own vehicle with hand controls, can drive independently, and pride myself on my reliability and punctuality." Another strategy in handling a blunt or stereotypical question, e.g., "I don't see how a cripple can do this job," would be to answer the intent of the question, i.e., how you will be able to do the job with your mobility problems. The response can then be framed to answer the concern and to make clear that you are capable of doing the job and performing the necessary tasks.

Reasonable Accommodations

The Americans with Disabilities Act (ADA) defines reasonable accommodations as, ". . .changes to the work environment or the way in which tasks are customarily performed to enable an individual with a disability to enjoy equal employment opportunities" (ADA, Title I, 1991). As indicated by the ADA, only functional limitations that affect the essential job duties of a position are considered when making job accommodations. The reasonable accommodations concept generally applies to the job application process, work environment, and work benefits and privileges. It is interesting to note that the Job Accommodation Network has reported that the average accommodation cost is less than $100 for the employer.

Ergonomic principles help fit the job to the person rather than make the person fit the job. For individuals with post-polio syndrome, the job accommodations discussed below improve opportunities to succeed in the workplace.

Accessible Workplace Facilities

Accessible workplace facilities are necessary if you have difficulty walking or climbing stairs, or if you use a wheelchair for mobility. Accessibility to workplace facilities is a primary consideration when contemplating employment. Often, the accommodations are not costly and can be explored through appropriate resources prior to an employment interview. Depending upon the specific job, company, and work site, the VR counselor can assist in educating the employer. Examples of modifications that employers may make include:

- Reserving extra-wide parking spaces near the building entrance
- Removing walkway obstructions
- Ramping stairways
- Regrading entranceways
- Widening entrance doorways
- Installing automatic door openers or lever doorknobs
- Installing elevators with lowered controls
- Providing accessible restrooms, lunchrooms, and training areas
- Leaving floors bare or installing low-pile carpeting.

Modified Work Schedules

Modified work schedules are simple, yet often overlooked, accommodations. An employer may be able to offer you a flexible work schedule by:

- Splitting the work position into multiple part-time jobs (also known as job-sharing)
- Adjusting work hours to reduce commuting time
- Allowing short, frequent rest breaks to encourage muscle recovery and to refresh concentration.

Job Restructuring

Job restructuring is an appropriate accommodation for almost any functional limitation you may experience. In job restructuring, nonessential functions are modified or reassigned to another employee in exchange for a task you can perform more easily. Examples of restructuring within a job might include:

- More telephone work instead of frequent travel
- Computerizing records instead of writing
- Rescheduling morning tasks to the afternoon or vice versa.

A real estate agent who has difficulty writing contracts, demonstrates this job restructuring principle when she executes property searches on a computer, while her colleague completes the written contracts.

Modified Workstations

Modified workstations contribute to the conservation of energy. Your workstation should be evaluated to determine the need for modification. Ask your VR counselor to suggest a rehabilitation engineer who may be available to make these modifications. Although some of the modifications may require the purchase of new items, many can be made with only minimal changes to existing equipment, including:

- Rearrange files or shelves to conserve energy
- Purchase a desktop turntable organizer to keep items within easy reach
- Organize your desk for face-to-face communication
- Relocate the desk to the most accessible area
- Raise and lower the desk to ensure proper seating posture; the desktop should be about an inch below your elbows
- Adjust the height of your computer screen to avoid neck and eye strain; the top of the computer screen should be at eye level
- Utilize a telephone headset.

Getting the Accommodations You Need

Most employers have policies and procedures for requesting accommodations. Again, this process begins with a written request, even if the discussion has occurred beforehand. You should use your own adaptive equipment whenever possible and keep solutions as simple and as cost-effective as possible. As a new applicant, you can request to tour the work area, observe the job being performed, and/or review the essential job requirements with the employer. In assessing this information, you (with or without the assistance of a VR counselor) can then submit a proposal for resources. This process can even be turned into a demonstration of your problem-solving skills.

In negotiating for the accommodations, you must be sensitive to the employer's perspective. You should present a rationale for its need as it relates to a specific job function. Again, do not assume that the employer has had any experience in this process. You must have a clear understanding of why the accommodation is needed and what benefit it has for the employer so that there will be less resistance. If architectural barrier changes are needed, the employer can be advised of the tax credits available for this purpose and how removal of the barriers may also potentially increase business.

Another strategy in handling employer's resistance is to make a referral to the Job Accommodation Network (JAN), an international, nonprofit information and referral service providing free consultation for accommodation needs, products, and services based in West Virginia. JAN provides information on accommodations to employers, especially on cost and resources. Employers can discuss options with the JAN staff and with other employers who have used the service. This service is provided at no cost to the employer. If a request for the provision of accommodations is denied, advocacy services can be obtained through a local center for independent living and vocational rehabilitation agencies.

Acquire the Assistive Devices You Need

When considering equipment to purchase, remember that the assistance device should address the functional limitation in that specific task. You may find the following helpful:

- Telephone headsets
- Electric scissors
- Anti-glare computer screens
- Ergonomic arm supports for forearm and wrist support while typing
- Tape recorders
- Dictaphones
- Voice-activated computers (The technology continues to improve and prices are dropping. Dragon Dictate® sells for under $200 and can recognize normal conversational speech.)
- Electric staplers.

Consider Job Relocation

Another option to consider is a change in the work environment. If you have mobility impairment or require special energy conservation techniques, changing to another more accessible location may be the possibility to pursue. Your treating physician may recommend this option. Documentation from your treating physician may be useful when discussing this option with human resources personnel. The VR counselor can assist in coordinating this effort. Some relocation options may include:

- Working at the company office closest to public transportation
- Working at home with a computer and modem connecting you to the office
- Changing the job location from the central office to a satellite office closer to your home
- Changing floors or work area location at the same site.

Retraining or Reassignment

Starting a new career path may be the best choice if you are unable to resume your current tasks, even with reasonable accommodations. As outlined in the ADA, your employer should provide the necessary retraining as long as it does not cause "an undue hardship" to the business. ADA states, "A current worker with a disability is eligible to be reassigned to those jobs for which s/he is qualified to perform. The only alternate placement positions to be considered are those that are currently vacant, or will be vacant within a reasonable amount of time."

Here are two examples of job accommodations. First, a librarian with post-polio who now must use a wheelchair is reassigned from the third floor to a similar position on the first floor. The building does not have an elevator, and it would be an "undue hardship" for the business to install one. Second, a legal secretary, who also answered phones and scheduled appointments, was unable to sustain eight hours of work at one time. A computer station was set up at home together with a change of duties involving more computer research, less typing, and no phone answering.

THE SCHOOL ACCOMMODATION PROCESS

If you are currently involved in an educational program, or if you anticipate enrolling, the school accommodation process can smooth the way. Community and four-year colleges, as well as vocational trade schools, are required to provide evidence that they accommodate disabled students. Guidance and counseling departments usually house the offices that manage disability programs. Many public/state higher learning institutions have a specific *Enabler* working with students and with the school.

As a student, you are responsible for initiating contact and requesting the specific assistance you need, such as:

- Tutorial services and readers
- Class note-takers
- Assistance in pushing a wheelchair
- Assistance with personal care.

The school can also make adjustments to the classroom environment. With some prior investigation on your part with the counseling department or the enabler, you can create a proactive plan to make the best use of academic opportunities. You may want to:

- Change a classroom site to an accessible area, particularly if there is no elevator in the building
- Ask that classroom seating be modified for easier wheelchair access
- Choose class times that coincide with your times of high energy
- Request oral exams and reports rather than written ones.

If you find resistance on the part of the school, request a meeting with a dean or another school official. If the resistance persists, seek help from your local advocacy group.

—11—

Navigating the Managed Care Maze

NAOMI NAIERMAN

Fast rising health-care costs have led the major payers, employers and government agencies to consider alternatives to the traditional fee-for-service health insurance system. In this system, doctors, hospitals, and other providers are reimbursed for services rendered with few restrictions and little scrutiny. Managed care, the increasingly more common alternative, is a system in which financial reimbursement is based on close review of medical decisions and on incentives rewarding providers with low-cost practice patterns.

The definition of managed care is still evolving. Broadly defined, it is an organized system of health-care delivery and financing designed to conserve resources. Its objectives are to minimize duplication, reduce inappropriate and unnecessary services, and substitute less expensive services. At its best, managed care emphasizes prevention and minimizes inefficiencies; at its worst, it constricts medical decisions and rations resources primarily for economic ends.

Above all, managed care is health insurance and, as such, it is governed by powerful incentives to minimize financial risk. Thus, it is safe to say, a managed care company prefers to sign up healthy persons, rather than sick people or people who need many services. Indeed, it is not uncommon to find marketing strategies specifically designed to attract healthy customers. Television ads for managed care companies reveal the ideal kinds of people they hope to attract: healthy, often young, people who are unlikely to need health services, except perhaps occasionally.

With the exponential growth of managed care, it behooves all of us to become more informed consumers. Certainly this is true for persons with post-polio, for no one is more vulnerable to the worst kinds of managed practices than people with chronic conditions because they are considered high risks by insurance companies. These practices include outright rejection of persons with prior conditions; higher charges levied against groups that include persons considered high-risk; and restriction of referrals to specialty services. To navigate through the managed care system, it is helpful to understand the features that shape physician behavior and the differences among major managed care models.

MANAGED CARE AND POST-POLIO

Managed care companies bring together consumers (often referred to as members) and providers (mainly physicians and hospitals). Members are encouraged to use network providers exclusively; opting outside the network means heavy financial penalties. In this way, providers are guaranteed the customers they need without the marketing and administrative responsibilities of recruiting and enrolling patients. In return, providers agree to a set of rules, including a monitoring system that reviews their practices and financial arrangements that reward low rates of utilization of such services as hospital admissions, referrals to specialists, and orders for lab tests and X-rays.

Whether physicians are hired as employees or engaged on a contractual basis, their medical practices are managed in a number of ways, including physician prescreening, utilization review, prior-authorization, gatekeeping, capitation, case management, and clinical practice guidelines. Each of these will be described briefly below, as they are important in understanding how physicians behave in a managed care system.

Prescreening

Before entering into a relationship with physicians, many managed care companies first prescreen (review) their pattern of providing services. These companies do so in order to identify cost-conscious physicians among all physicians in the same specialty. Do they have a higher hospital admission rate than their peers? Do they order more X-rays or laboratory tests on the average for a given condition? Do they refer to specialists more often?

It is not uncommon for physicians with patterns far exceeding the norm to be avoided by managed care companies, even if their practices are explained by a disproportionately large number of very sick people. In other words, physicians who serve many persons with disabilities may not be attractive to managed care companies because they bring with them a panel of individuals who are considered high-risk by insurance standards. The potential effect is to discourage physicians from treating persons with a chronic condition such as post-polio.

Utilization Review

Almost all managed care companies employ a utilization review process by which every physician is scrutinized for the number and reasons for certain high-cost services. The average for an individual physician is compared to the average of all the others employed or contracted by the company. Deviations from the overall average are treated in a variety of ways, including simple reminders, requests for explanations, financial rewards for those who fall below the average, financial penalties for those who do not, a series of warnings, and even dismissal from the approved network of providers. The effect of this scrutiny is to curb the number of tests and referrals ordered by physicians to keep their managed care jobs or contracts.

To the extent that some referrals and tests are unnecessary, the impact is minimal. On the other hand, restraint imposed on physicians does not bode well for persons who rely on multiple physicians or on an array of procedures. Intense scrutiny combined with attractive financial rewards may lead some physicians to make their clinical decisions, not on a medical basis, but rather on an economic basis. For post-polios, this economic basis may present a problem if they need many diagnostic tests or multiple interventions to address their various symptoms.

Prior Authorization

Aside from monitoring the quantity and costs of medical practices, a managed care company may require prior approval of certain recommendations that doctors make. Except in an emergency, most hospital admissions and surgical procedures require a prior authorization, as do very expensive procedures.

It is not uncommon for managed care companies to limit the number of physical therapy sessions and many other specialty services that persons with chronic conditions may need. Nor is it uncommon for certain treatments to be disallowed from reimbursement altogether, when they are considered costly and optional. Rehabilitation treatments may be regarded as dispensable, especially when there is little documentation about the difference they make on a person's health. Even with evidence about their benefits, however, the nature and intensity of rehabilitation services reimbursed under managed care are functions of economic consideration that vary among managed care plans.

Gatekeeping

In certain types of managed care plans, members are encouraged to choose a single primary care physician, most often an internist, family physician, or pediatrician. This physician is assigned the responsibility of coordinating the care of the member, acting as the gatekeeper to other services. The gatekeeping role, required by some, though not all, managed care companies, means that a member cannot seek any other care without a referral from the gatekeeping physician.

In most managed care plans, gatekeeping physicians are financially rewarded for keeping their referrals low. The funds usually come from a pool set aside for reimbursing specialists or providers of ancillary services (e.g., X-rays). If there is any money left in the pool, the low-cost gatekeeping physicians get rewarded, and the high cost physicians do not.

This practice does not serve the interests of persons with post-polio, unless there is a gatekeeping physician with expertise in post-polio. If, in addition, there is a need for specialty services, it is important to find out how readily accessible these services are within the gatekeeping confines.

Capitation

Primary care physicians in managed care organizations are often paid on a per-capita basis. Capitation is a monthly payment made by the managed care company to a physician for each member in his or her panel. The same amount is paid, regardless of how often the members are served. The fewer the visits, the higher the physician's profits. This system does not reward doctors who welcome many visits by their patients. Since post-polio individuals are likely to need multiple visits with their primary care physician, it is important to determine to what extent capitation shapes the behavior of the doctor under consideration.

Clinical Practice Guidelines

Increasingly, more managed care companies have developed clinical practice guidelines that are evidence-based instructions for physicians. They are usually developed for the treatment of persons with certain high-volume and/or high-cost conditions, such as diabetes and asthma.

Because post-polio does not readily fall into this category, it is unlikely that specific clinical practice guidelines will be devised. Yet, the mere presence of such guidelines in a managed care plan raises a question about the way medical practice is monitored. On the one hand, these guidelines help doctors make better informed decisions; on the other hand, they can be used to generate a cookie-cutter approach to care. This means that individual considerations and unique circumstances may be overlooked to give way to standardized treatment plans.

TYPES OF MANAGED CARE

There are hundreds of managed care plans sprouting throughout the country and there is yet no standard topology to describe them. From a consumer's perspective, it is practical to focus on the three generic types: preferred provider organization (PPO); health maintenance organization (HMO), and point of services (POS) organization. A fourth type, medical or disease management, is emerging as a new approach to address chronic disease populations, including persons with disabilities. Each of these types will be described below.

Preferred Provider Organizations (PPOs)

Preferred provider organizations (PPOs) are designed to reduce health-care costs through volume discounts. In return for a critical mass of members, PPOs exact reduced fees from physicians, hospitals, and other providers. For their part, PPO members can keep their out-of-pocket costs low, if they use PPO providers. Insurance coverage is also available for services provided outside the PPO provider panel, but at a much reduced level.

In PPOs, there is little scrutiny or coordination of physician practices, although certain high-cost services require prior authorization. Physicians do not assume a gatekeeping role, nor do they share financial risk through capitation. Physicians with high rates of referrals and utilization patterns are less likely to be invited to join PPOs than those with more conservative practice patterns.

PPOs offer more choice among providers and more freedom of movement among specialists than alternative managed care models. Since PPOs impose few if any restrictions on referrals, members are free to go from one physician to another without prior approval. Therefore, for persons who rely on more than one physician, the PPO alternative may be advisable. Since PPO physicians are not rewarded for less care and fewer referrals, the PPO model may also be suitable for those who require ongoing therapy, tests, and other procedures

In return for these relatively flexible benefits, consumers should expect to spend more in premiums, deductibles, and copayments than they would under other managed care models. There is also the burden of claims filing, although it is much reduced compared to traditional insurance.

Health Maintenance Organizations (HMOs)

To keep their cost low and to minimize their financial risk, HMOs use most, if not all, of the available cost control mechanisms. Prescreening, utilization review, and prior authorizations are universal among HMOs. Gatekeeping and capitation are also common in HMOs, while clinical practice guidelines are found more sporadically. In HMOs, physicians operate under considerable scrutiny, which may have an impact on their clinical decisions. They may also be affected by financial rewards that invariably favor fewer services and referrals.

For their part, HMO members are confined exclusively to the HMO panel of providers; opting outside the network usually means no reimbursement for services rendered. On the other hand, the deductibles and copayments in an HMO are lower when compared to PPO charges. Indeed, many HMOs require no copayments. These low, out-of-pocket costs are especially important for persons who need to see a doctor on a regular basis. Finally, HMOs relieve the members of all claim filing, so there is virtually no paperwork required.

HMOs fall into two major types: 1) the staff model, in which all physicians are employees paid on a salary basis; and 2) the independent practice association (IPA), which contract with office-based physicians, most of whom work with a number of HMOs. The difference between these models is that, while both monitor physicians closely, the referrals to specialists may not be as restricted in the staff model HMOs. Since some, though not all, specialists are HMO employees, their services are already being paid by the staff model HMO. Depending on the number of specialists and the demand for their services, they may not create extra expenses.

In contrast, referrals in an IPA are more likely to generate extra costs, which are often subtracted from the bonus pool set aside for physicians. The more referrals that IPA physicians make, the less money they get from this pool. Another difference is that staff model HMOs have centralized facilities, whereas IPA physicians are, by definition, spread out geographically. For persons with post-polio, the geographic location may be an important feature of convenience.

Point of Service (POS)

Point of service (POS) managed care plans are hybrid HMOs that leave the gate partially open to traditional insurance coverage. Members may opt to use services outside the HMO but not without financial penalties. The premiums are higher and the deductibles can be quite steep. When using the out-of-panel providers, members are required to file claims forms.

The POS option has become popular of late, especially among large employers or employer coalitions that can negotiate more reasonable premium rates than their smaller counterparts. It is popular because it offers more choice, allowing enrollees to select virtually any physician or hospital. With this option, an individual with post-polio syndrome is not completely locked into a panel of physicians. This panel may not include post-polio specialists, however, so the cost of using experts outside the HMO panel of physicians could be prohibitive.

Disease Management

Rather than limiting access to specialists, this model of managed care uses certain specialists as primary providers and gatekeepers for certain high-cost diseases or conditions. This approach has been developed by managed care companies to coordinate the care of the very sick, who account for a disproportionate amount of the health-care costs.

Traditionally, health insurance companies try to keep this very sick population out of their pools. Recently, large investments have been made in information systems, clinical practice guidelines, and other medical systems necessary to detect and manage the populations that use most of the health-care resources. After only a few years of a research and development phase, it is already clear that certain conditions, such as diabetes and asthma, can be better managed from both a medical and an economic perspective. This approach seems promising for persons with post-polio, if it is implemented by physicians who are knowledgeable about the condition.

BE YOUR OWN CAPTAIN

To navigate effectively through the managed care maze, be prepared to be your own captain. Based on your initial polio experience, you have probably mastered the art of being your own advocate and you have also learned how important it is to inform yourself about your condition and your needs. This experience will serve you well, if you are to find your way through the managed care maze.

Start with as much knowledge as you can gather about managed care, about post-polio in general, and about your own particular version. This book is designed to arm you with state-of-the-art information about post-polio and some of the most pertinent information about managed care. Find a doctor with expertise in post-polio. A local polio support group is a good source for such a referral, should you need one. If it is difficult to find a physician with post-polio expertise in your community, find one who is willing to learn. Whether or not your preferred doctor knows about post-polio, he/she should read this book.

Next, identify the managed care plan(s) that your chosen doctor belongs to. Hopefully, you will have access to these plans through your employer or on your own. If your employer offers other plans, lobby for your own choice of physician or shop for a compatible physician among the plans available to you.

If you have a choice among several types of managed care plans, pick one that affords flexibility with respect to referrals. Some are less rigid than others. The most advanced plans allow a specialist to play the gatekeeping role for certain conditions, thus removing the need to see a primary care physician first. If you can afford the higher out-of-pocket costs, consider a point-of-service (POS) plan, if it is available to you. It will afford you the option of going to virtually any specialist, should you need one in the future.

Look for a managed care plan that has generous physical therapy, occupational therapy, home health care, and other kinds of specific services that you may need now or in the future. If these are not spelled out, ask at the member services department, or even better, track down current members and inquire about their actual experience in getting needed services.

Should you find yourself being challenged by the managed care plan with respect to needed services, you have at least three courses. First, try engaging your physician as your advocate. If this does not go far enough with the managed care plan, be prepared to make your own case by making lots of calls at various levels of the organization until you get the desired response. As a last resort, call the state insurance company and register a complaint. Legal action may be appropriate when all else fails and when legal advice points in that direction.

12

Playing the Social Security Benefits Card

KATHRYN R. B. MCGOWAN

Persons with post-polio syndrome strive to maintain financial independence, yet this goal becomes difficult to achieve when you are experiencing new physical limitations or conserving energy. As a consequence, many persons dealing with post-polio syndrome face reductions in work income or even in their ability to work at all. The Social Security Administration sponsors two programs that offer means of financial assistance which may help individuals balance goals of financial independence with the demands of post-polio syndrome. One program provides Social Security Disability Insurance (SSDI), and the other offers Supplemental Security Income (SSI).

SSDI differs from SSI in three very important ways: it is partially needs-based; it considers prior work experience as a factor in its eligibility determination; and its benefit payments begin from the date of disability onset. SSI is entirely needs-based; it is available to qualified individuals regardless of their prior work history; and its benefit payments begin from the date of application. The important thing to remember is that benefits are available, and there are resources to assist you financially and to keep you up-to-date with the most current policies and eligibility requirements. Resources are listed in the Appendix and are available at your local Social Security Administration office.

SOCIAL SECURITY DISABILITY INSURANCE (SSDI)

Similar to the Social Security Administration's retirement program, SSDI provides cash benefits to qualified individuals based upon their prior work experience which contributed taxable income towards the Social Security Administration. SSDI, however, has no age restrictions.

Qualification Criteria

The qualifications for SSDI benefits fall into two broad categories. The first has to do with your work history, and the second pertains to your disability status. To meet the work history eligibility criteria, you must have contributed to the Social Security Administration through your earnings for a certain number of years. The Social Security Administration measures years in terms of quarters, or work credits. It requires you to earn a certain amount of income per quarter in order to receive a work credit. The earnings value of a work credit increases yearly as the general wage rises. Depending upon whether or not you earn enough to receive a work credit, you can potentially acquire up to four work credits each year. The number of work credits you have to amass for SSDI eligibility status depends upon the age of disability onset.

The Social Security Administration defines disability as "The inability of a person to perform any substantial gainful activity by reason of a medically determinable physical or mental impairment which can be expected to result in death or has lasted, or can be expected to last, for a continuous period of not less than twelve consecutive months." Two phrases in this definition deserve clarification: "substantial gainful activity" and "can be expected . . . to last . . . not less than twelve consecutive months." Substantial gainful activity is any activity that generates an average of $500 or more each month. Any activity that produces less than an average of $300 per month is not considered substantial and gainful. An acknowledged gray area exists between $300 and $500. Brief intermittent periods of work do not count as substantial gainful activity.

There are a couple of misconceptions regarding substantial gainful activity which need to be dispelled. One misconception is that the earnings of the applicant's spouse are counted as substantial and gainful income. The Social Security Administration is only interested in the applicant's total worth—your spouse's income is not a factor in SSDI eligibility determination. Another misconception has to do with home ownership. The Social Security Administration does not count the portion of home ownership for which you have already paid as substantial and gainful income.

The disability qualifier, ". . . can be expected to last . . . not less than twelve consecutive months" depends upon a physician's judgment. It does not mean that you have to be disabled and unemployed for twelve continuous months before you can consider applying for SSDI. For example, a physician can confirm that you became disabled one month prior to filing an initial SSDI claim and that you are expected to remain disabled for the next eleven months after the claim is made.

Application and Appeals Process

Proof of a medically diagnosed disability is essential to the SSDI claims process—more so than evidence of your inability to work. The Social Security Administration does not provide SSDI to persons who are partially or temporarily disabled. To build a strong claim for disability, your medical history should document the following:

- A description of your original diagnosis of polio
- The degree of your original polio-related paralysis
- Descriptions of all new functional restrictions
- Onset of new problems, and related accommodations in activities of daily living
- Dates of treatments and names, addresses, and phone numbers of any clinician or institution which treated you through the years—not just those who most recently treated you.

The Social Security Administration will measure your case of polio-related disability against its definition of post-polio syndrome. The Social Security Administration catalogues all disabilities in its *Listing of Impairments*, and it lists post-polio syndrome as: "The claimant must provide competent medical evidence of Anterior Poliomyelitis as well as persistent difficulty with swallowing or breathing, unintelligible speech, or disorganization of motor function in two extremities resulting in sustained disturbance of gross and dexterous movements, or gait and station." The closer your medical history documents a case which corresponds to the Social Security

Administration's listing for post-polio syndrome, the stronger your claim will be.

In addition to your medical history, try to locate the following information to expedite your claim process:

- Social security card or record of the number
- Proof of age
- Documentation of your work history for the past fifteen years, including names and addresses of employers
- Documentation of income, including your W-2 if you were employed or your federal tax return if you were unemployed.

With these materials on hand, locate your nearest Social Security Administration office by calling 1-800-772-1213 and submit your claim. If you do not have all of your work-related materials available, your local Social Security Administration office can assist you in locating any necessary documents. Also, if the Social Security Administration finds your proof of disability inadequate, it will pay for any additional examinations and reports it requires.

Your local Social Security Administration office will forward your application to your state's Disability Determination Service (DDS). If the DDS denies your claim, you can request a reconsideration of their decision within sixty days of your rejection notification. If your claim continues to be denied, you can continue to request reconsiderations through four levels of administrative appeals and three levels of legal appeals that include filing civil suits in the Federal District Court, the Court of Appeals, and the U.S. Supreme Court. At each level, you have 60 days to file a reconsideration upon receiving a rejection notification.

To navigate the appeals processes, you may wish to hire an attorney who is knowledgeable about SSDI. It is said that 60 percent to 70 percent of applicants are turned down on their initial application. The advice of experienced lawyers in this area is to not get discouraged and to keep trying until you reach the third level of administrative appeals. Beyond this point and before pursuing civil suits, carefully consider the costs—both in time and in legal fees—these may outweigh any actual SSDI benefit received. For the story of one polio survivor's successful application for SSDI benefits, see Nancy Carter's personal testimony found in the last chapter in this book.

Payment of Benefits

If your claim for SSDI is approved, your payments will begin in the sixth full month after the onset of your disability. If the approval process takes longer than six months, checks are dated back to that month. The amount of your SSDI check is based on your lifetime average earnings that contributed taxable income. The amount may be reduced if you are eligible for or receive worker's compensation or any type of pension. You should be aware that, depending on your total income from all sources, including SSDI, you may have to pay federal income tax on these benefits. Finally, the SSDI program provides work incentives to its beneficiaries which enable them to work without losing their SSDI benefits. Discussion of these various work incentives exceeds the scope of this chapter, however, you can obtain detailed information from the Social Security Administration which specifically addresses the guidelines.

SUPPLEMENTAL SECURITY INCOME (SSI) FOR PERSONS WITH DISABILITIES

The Supplemental Security Income program provides a basic monthly income to persons who are aged 65 or older, blind, or permanently and totally disabled. Unlike SSDI, this basic monthly income is indexed according to an annually adjusted cost of living set by the federal government.

Qualification Criteria

As a general guideline, those who qualify for food stamps or for Medicaid will qualify for SSI benefits. Specifically, four categories of criteria determine whether or not you are eligible for SSI. First, you must be one of the following:

- Disabled from a physical or mental problem that keeps you from working for an expected period of one year or that will result in death
- Aged 65 or older
- Totally or very partially blind, regardless of age.

The second set of SSI criteria deals with residency. You must be an American citizen or a legal alien. Also, with few exceptions, applicants who live in city or county rest homes, halfway houses, or other public institutions do not qualify for SSI benefits.

The third category of criteria applies to items owned by individuals or couples applying for SSI. Qualified individuals cannot own items worth $2000 or more; a married couple of two eligible individuals cannot own $3000 or more. The calculation of worth includes real estate, bank accounts, cash, stocks, and bonds. Calculations do not include the worth of an applicant's home, the land on which a residence rests, or burial plots for an applicant or his/her immediate family. Calculations may or may not include personal or household goods, life insurance policies, cars, "up to but not including" $1500 in burial funds for an applicant and his/her spouse, and items potentially used towards work or education.

The fourth set of criteria addresses income. To be eligible for SSI, the Social Security Administration will consider as countable income social security checks, pensions, taxable earnings, and non-cash items such as food or clothing. The maximum amount of income an individual or couple can have and still qualify for SSI benefits depends on the state in which they live. To learn more about your state's SSI policies, call 1-800-772-1213.

Application Process

To expedite your application for SSI upon contacting your local Social Security Administration office, gather together the following information:

- Names, addresses, and phone numbers of clinicians and institutions who treated you for your disability
- Social security card or record of the number
- Proof of age
- Information about the ownership and financing of your home
- Payroll slips, bank books, insurance policies, car registrations, burial fund records, and other information documenting possessions and income.

As with SSDI, your local Social Security Office will help you locate all necessary documents if these are not readily available to you.

Payments of Benefits

If you are approved for SSI, you will receive a full monthly allotment during the second month of payment. The amount of your monthly SSI check will vary depending upon the state in which you live and your net monthly income. Whether or not a monthly SSI payment exceeds the base level amount set by the federal government depends upon the state in which the beneficiary lives. Some states add to this base level. Whether or not a monthly SSI payment is less than the base level amount depends upon your individual or family income generated each month. Like the SSDI program, you can work and continue to receive SSI payments provided that your average monthly income does not exceed SSI limits set for you. For details on the SSI's work incentive options, obtain the publication *Working While Disabled* from the Social Security Administration.

—13—

A Guide to the Internet for Polio Survivors

ANNE C. GAWNE
TOM WALTER

At the simplest level, the Internet is an interconnected network of computers all over the world, all linked together sharing information. Through the Internet, users in any location can send and receive electronic data, including text, pictures and sound. No central computer controls this network; instead, the Internet relies upon cooperation among a group of independent organizations.

The worldwide network is maintained by telephone lines, satellites, and microwaves. Three large switching stations, called network access points, are located in Chicago, San Francisco, and New York. The headquarters for metropolitan exchanges is located in Washington, D.C. The main guidance and coordination are provided by the Internet Society (ISOC). The ISOC helps develop and maintain the "rules of the road."

A SHORT HISTORY OF THE INTERNET

The Internet began development on January 2, 1969, when the Advanced Research Project Agency of the Department of the Defense (DOD) linked together four computers in universities in California and Utah. Electronic mail (E-mail) was developed in 1972 to deliver mail across a network of 40 computers. By 1977, the number was up to 100 host computers. The DOD added Milnet for military activities in 1982. When the two networks combined, the term Internet was created to describe this connection. Services included E-mail, list-serves, and search features, which included primarily text. At that time, the Internet was based on a computer language known as UNIX, which was limited largely to the scientific community. By 1984, the number of computers had expanded to 1000, mainly at universities and military agencies. The National Science Foundation (NSF) assumed responsibility for the Internet in 1986, expanding the backbone of central computers to 13 sites in the United States and increasing the speed of processing over the network. Until 1991, the Internet was restricted to military, education, research, and nonprofit activities. In that year, commercial activities were allowed for the first time. In the following year, the World Wide Web (WWW) was begun.

In 1992, a programmer named Tim Berners-Lee established a protocol that permitted one to point and click while on the Internet to gain access to text and graphics on the World Wide Web. Corporations, companies, nonprofit organizations, and even the White House began to create Web Home Pages to offer information about their services, products, or purposes. More than 10 million computers were on the Internet throughout the United States and in countries worldwide in early 1997.

RESOURCES AVAILABLE ON THE INTERNET

Electronic Mail

E-mail allows Internet users to communicate directly with each other. Each user has a distinct address usually designated by some combination of the user's name or initials, then the "at" sign @, the institution or Internet Service Provider (ISP) followed by a dot, and closing with the type of institution (i.e., your name@*ISP.com*). In this case, *com* stands for commercial provider, but other identifying extensions include *edu* for education, *gov* for government and *org* for organization.

Mailing Lists

Mailing lists are a form of E-mail where everyone on the mailing list receives the same message. Anyone with similar interests can communicate this way without having to send separate messages. Usually one person is in charge of maintaining the mailing list and updating it, adding and subtracting names as people join or leave the list, reminding members to stay on the subject and use good electronic manners, and keeping people off the list who do not qualify for membership. One major type of mail list is known as LISTSERV.

Newsgroups

Newsgroups are a forum for exchange of information on a certain topic. They are similar to a bulletin board service and are frequently updated. To access a newsgroup, one can use a browser included with the ISP's software. The advantage of a newsgroup is that it provides wide dissemination of publicly accessible information. Some disadvantages are that news systems will expire and may not always be updated. Newsgroups are also usually not moderated. The Usenet Newsgroup for PPS is alt.support.post-polio.

The World Wide Web

Web sites are designated by an address called a Uniform Resource Locator (URL), such as—*http://www.whitehouse.gov*. Governmental, educational, organizational and commercial web sites offer visual, audio, and video presentations of information.

File Transfer Protocol

This service offers a way to transfer large files of information from one user to another. For instance, you can use it to log on to access files in public libraries, the Library of Congress, and the National Library of Medicine. Programs are available through the WWW or an ISP, but many times passwords are needed to gain access. This service is not as commonly used as it was just a few short years ago.

NETIQUETTE

Netiquette is a set of guidelines to facilitate use of the Internet for everyone. These "rules of the road" include:

- Read before posting
- Read the "frequently asked questions" (FAQ) file before asking a question
- Avoid sending derogatory remarks, swearing, or using offensive language
- Avoid flame wars or getting into arguments on the Net
- Use humor carefully; the written word does not always convey humor reliably
- Humor can be used if "smileys" or "emoticons" (symbols that display emotion) are added
- Avoid trolling, purposely inflammatory or annoying posts
- Avoid cascading; cascading occurs when one decides to get in the last word
- Avoid degrading gossip or comments
- Avoid temptation to crosspost messages from one list to another
- In responding to a message, avoid resending the original message. Use just enough of the original message to convey context or subject
- Avoid using technical language and acronyms whenever possible unless the meaning of the acronym is included within the original message
- TYPING IN CAPITAL LETTERS should be avoided; use asterisks or underline for emphasis
- Check for proper spelling and grammar
- Always sign messages with your name and E-mail address.

PRIVACY AND SAFEGUARDS

Those not familiar with the Internet should be aware that when you post a message to a message board, it can be accessed by virtually anyone with a computer. Therefore, it's not wise to give out personal information or identification, such as an address or a telephone number (except in private E-mail to someone you know).

EQUIPMENT AND SOFTWARE

The best way to become familiar with the Internet is to learn from someone who already is set up and has the necessary equipment and skills. Then, make the decision if the Internet is something you really want to pursue and have the necessary time, energy, and money. Although the computer revolution is here to stay, it isn't for everyone and you shouldn't feel obliged to join if you don't want to participate. There will always be plenty of people willing to show you what they can do and share what they have learned.

If you want to get your own computer or upgrade the computer you have to access the Internet, you will need to become an informed consumer. Many options are available, and you will need to make a number of decisions depending on your interests and desires. Also, innumerable resources exist to help you make those decisions: friends, books, magazines, and, ultimately, the companies that market the products.

An ISP is a company like America Online (AOL) that provides access to the Internet through local phone lines. To find an ISP, look in the yellow pages and your local paper, or ask colleagues or friends. A good ISP should offer access through a local or 1-800 phone line. The ISP should offer unlimited time for about $20/month. Services should include E-mail, a fast connection, accessible technical support, and up-to-date software.

Search engines are programs that allow you to look for specific information. Search engines include programs such as YAHOO, Infoseek, Lycos, Excite, and Alta Vista. When you first access Internet software such as Netscape Navigator or Microsoft Internet Explorer, sometimes search engine choices will appear on the screen.

POST-POLIO RESOURCES ON THE WEB

The following discussion provides a brief overview for post-polio survivors on the resources to be found on the Internet. Several of these are available on the World Wide Web. One chat group is described for interaction with other post-polios and as sources for new information. Finally, instructions for subscribing to the Internet polio mailing list are provided. The mailing list is also a great way to exchange information and find support from other survivors.

WWW Information Home Pages

Four WWW information home pages are described below.

The Lincolnshire Post-Polio Network site can be found at the following WWW home page address:—*http://www.zynet.co.uk/ott/polio/lincolnshire/*. It is maintained by the post-polio support group in Lincolnshire, England, and is a good place to start your search for information. Resources include a library of up-to-date articles, medical information, and general facts about PPS.

The P.R.Y.S. (Polio—Remember YOUR Strength). This nonprofit private foundation's site includes polio web site links, medical information, poems, stories, and books of interest. *http://www.prys.net/home.html*

Rollin' Rat Web Page.—*http://www.azstarnet.com/~rspear/* This home page includes articles on post-polio fatigue and how it can change your mind and much, much more.

The Polio Survivors Page.—(*http://www.eskimo.com/~dempt/polio.html*) This home page includes announcements, articles, a post-polio information packet, newsletters, and other resources.

Chat Groups

Each Tuesday at 9:30pm ET, polio survivors who are also AOL members meet for fellowship and discussion of post-polio syndrome symptoms, diagnosis, and treatment for one hour at the Equal Access Café. Logs of previous meetings with text of the conversation are made available for downloading and reading off-line by requesting them from *tomincal@AOL.com.*

Mailing Lists

The Internet polio mailing list was started in September 1994 for the purpose of exchanging information and support and providing fellowship among polio survivors, their friends, and relatives. Each message posted is automatically distributed as E-mail to all other subscribers. To subscribe, send an E-mail message from the account where you wish to receive mail to *listserv@maelstrom.stjohns.edu* with a message in the first line only of the body, reading: *sub polio yourfirstname yourlastname*.

HINTS FOR USING THE INTERNET

Hints for using the Internet are as follows:

- To start with, get some help from someone experienced in using the Net
- Be ready to waste some time "surfing" from place to place as a good way to learn
- Spend some time before you go "online" getting comfortable with the function of the mouse and other keys on the computer
- Call your ISP if you need technical help
- Have patience while connections are made as you go from site to site
- As with any skill, practice makes perfect, so the more time you spend on the Net, the better you will be at using it
- As you spend more time on the Net, upgrade your equipment as your pocketbook allows
- Caveat emptor (buyer beware): in this case, Internet user beware. The quality and accuracy of information on the Net varies enormously from scientific articles in prestigious, peer-reviewed journals to gossip from the next-door neighbor
- Finally, have fun, learn things, and make friends!!

Appendix: Personal Stories

Polio Memories from the Class of 1952 and Maturing with Polio

Joyce Ann Tepley

My brother and I got polio in 1952, one of the last epidemic summers in the United States. I was nine years old and he was a baby. The virus left him with very little use of his right arm. My back and legs were paralyzed. That first dark night in the isolation hospital ward still haunts me. I felt sick with flu-like symptoms, was sore from the spinal tap, and was too scared to cry. I can still hear the other children crying just before I finally drifted off to sleep. The next morning I could not even lift my head from the pillow. My life seemed far away from only the day before when I was riding my bicycle around the block.

Looking back on 1951BP (Before Polio), my life seemed ideal. I felt safe and loved, I was having fun, the new school experience was good, and my body worked. Now, sometimes at night before I fall asleep, I try to conjure up the feelings I had at that time. I try to re-experience in my mind what it was like to take off running when my friend, Eddy, started chasing me as the sheriff and I was Black Bart. It amazes me now that I was not afraid of tripping and falling. I can remember feeling so proud of what my body could do, making my parents watch me over and over do leg splits and back bends. I went to dancing school when I was seven and eight, and loved showing off my graceful steps.

It was an innocent time. My parents protected me from the stresses they were experiencing. My father was trying to make a go of his own business, a small tool and die machine shop. We just had a new addition to the family, my brother. They bought a house for the first time in their marriage with the help of my mother's parents. They were in debt but hopeful of a new life of prosperity, like so many couples after the war. I never knew the fear they must have felt, because they demonstrated that, in order to live well, you have to take chances and trust in yourself. Taking chances that year included going to summer day camp when the city was held hostage by the poliovirus. I am sure they were afraid for me, like hundreds of other parents were, but they also knew how important it was for me to have my first camping experience. We speculated later that I must have gotten the poliovirus from day camp and brought it home to my brother.

I will never forget that life-altering day in July. Sometime during the early afternoon I started feeling sick to my stomach and feverish. It felt like I was getting the flu. My mother called Dr. Cassidy, our kindly, gray-haired family doctor. He said he would be at our house as soon as he could. Doctors still made house calls at that time, and Dr. Cassidy knew my family well. By the time he got there I was very weak. He took one look at me and told my parents to take me to City Hospital emergency room immediately. No one mentioned the dreaded word, polio, as I stumbled into the car. The next thing I remember was lying curled up on my side under a harsh light while a nurse held me for the doctor to stick a needle in my back. I was very scared, but the nurse's touch and kind words of reassurance helped me endure having to lie very still with a needle in my back. So far, this was the worst thing that had ever happened to me. Little did I realize what more was to come.

After the doctor was finished with his test they let my parents see me. Mom and Dad looked very worried when they told me I would have to stay in the hospital for a while. I do not remember when I first knew that I got polio. I just remember how drastically my body changed. I did not know what to expect. I must have heard stories of other children who got polio, but I did not pay attention and all my friends were healthy like me. Some days went by before my parents were allowed to see me again. I had spent time away from home visiting girlfriends since I was six years old, but that was fun. This time being in an unfamiliar place was frightening, and I could hardly move. I also did not know that my parents brought my brother to the hospital a few days after me. He was in intensive care being observed for bulbar polio. After the life-threatening crisis was over, they were able to take him home with physical therapy instructions. He was eight months old. They had their hands full.

The acute stage treatment at the hospital was rest, "hot packs" and splints. I had to wear the metal and felt-lined splints all the time so that my leg muscles would not draw up. The splints would not allow me to turn over, and they were very itchy. I was so thankful when Mom brought me a wooden back scratcher so I could get inside the felt lining and scratch my legs. Twice a day an old ringer washing machine was brought into the ward from which the nurses administered the "hot pack" treatment. Some children cried. When my turn came the nurse opened the lid of the machine, reached inside with her long tongs, pulled out a steaming strip of army green blanket and put it through the wringer. Then she pulled back my covers and laid the strip on my leg. She covered all my limbs with hot strips and put the blanket over me. When the strips cooled she came back and removed them. After the initial fear that I would be burned, it was actually a comforting experience. I later learned that my brother's arm was accidentally burned from this treatment. My parents were livid.

The "instruments of medical torture" were frightening, but I endured them bravely because the hope was held out to me that I would overcome the disease. My arms seemed to be unaffected by the paralysis. I could still move them after my fever broke and I started feeling better. However, in those first couple weeks, I could not sit up or move my legs no matter how hard I tried. My parents were told not to expect me to walk again, but they didn't let me know that. They kept encouraging me to try and held out the hope that I would get better.

I remember how triumphant I felt a few weeks later when I could raise my head from the bed. How proud they were of me when I showed them what I could do the next time they came to see me. It was like showing off for them when I was in dancing school; only for them it must have been more poignant. Shortly afterward I was able to sit up in a chair for short periods of time. It was exhausting. I comforted myself with the knowledge that I was luckier than some of the friends I had made in the hospital who would have to live permanently in an iron lung. I felt homesick and lonesome for my old friends.

After a long two months, I was transferred to a residential children's rehabilitation facility called Rainbow Hospital, an hour's drive from our home. The strain on my parents of the long drive was an enormous sacrifice in time and effort. At that time I had no idea how difficult the whole ordeal was for them, but they did not want me to feel neglected. They were always encouraging, never showing the fear they must have had that I would not be able to walk again. I often wonder how they kept from going crazy during those first nightmarish months. Over the years I have received much recognition for what I have been able to do with my life "despite my disability," but the unsung heroes are my parents.

If I had been younger I might have felt more abandoned, but since I was at that stage in my childhood development when independence is tested and friends are more important than family, I adjusted well to group living with my peers. I definitely looked forward, though, to the weekend visits from my parents when I could tell them all the things I did during the week. Sometimes they would bring Grandma and she would bring her wonderful fried chicken. They would wheel me outside in my iron-barred bed, and we would have a picnic. I remember them bringing me a portable radio with a dial for tuning my favorite stations. I have only a few photographs of my nine months' stay at Rainbow. One of them is of me lying in my bed on my stomach, raised up by my elbows, showing off a prick on my finger from a recent blood test. The radio was right next to me. My parents always took lots of pictures as we were growing up. I wonder why they only took a few during that time? Perhaps it was a time too painful to record.

Living at Rainbow was mostly a good experience. The tree-lined grounds were very pretty, and the heated indoor pool was great to exercise in, though I don't remember ever using the pool just for fun. Life settled into a busy routine of sleeping, eating, physical therapy, and school. I started fourth grade there in the Fall so I wouldn't get behind in my studies. I didn't have time to be homesick. I developed a close friendship with Maryann, a girl in the bed next to mine who also had polio. We were the same age so we played, and giggled, and talked a lot. We were in a big brightly lit wing with lots of windows and many beds. I think there were curtains between all the beds, but I don't remember much privacy. Even though I was a little shy, I could make friends easily. However, I preferred to always have a best friend and Maryann was it for my time at Rainbow.

The nurses and therapists were generally nice but understandably tough. I tried to be a "good girl," having had Catholic guilt instilled in me very early in my education. I wanted to please the staff and my parents. I did everything I was told to do. I was working hard to recover whatever muscle strength I had left. I was fitted with long leg braces and, as I got stronger, I used the wheelchair less and less. I learned to fall down and get up without help. I learned to climb steps. Painful hours were spent stretching my hamstrings. There was little room for feelings of frustration, anger, or fear. I had learned enough discipline at home and school to bear any discomfort in order to reach my goal. One day as one of the physical therapists was enthusiastically stretching my ankle under water, she accidentally sprained it. I remember how much it hurt, but I didn't complain because the goal was set for me to walk again without braces or my two canes. I was never shamed for needing to use them. It was just expected that if I worked hard enough, I would simply not need them someday.

Being good and being brave was a tall order for a little girl. I did a great job of suppressing any "bad" feelings. I also had plenty of help in that endeavor. One of the nurses who had night duty was a favorite of Maryann's and mine. She was short, had red hair, and would read us Raggedy Ann stories at bedtime. I liked her because she made us feel special. One night, however, I got angry about something and couldn't stop myself from throwing a temper tantrum. I yelled at her in full rebellion. I will never forget how swiftly she dealt with me by yanking my heavy bed out of the ward, and rolling me into a small room isolating me until I calmed down. I was mortified. I was also helpless to protest any further. I never did *that* again. Soon she came to ask me if I was ready to go back to the ward. She wasn't angry with me, but I was very concerned about disappointing her and spoiling the way she thought of me as a "good little girl."

Christmas was coming and the hospital was putting up decorations. We had a big tree in the ward with lots of wrapped presents under it. One of the gifts was a big box and I remember looking yearningly at it every day. Some of us would be lucky enough to go home for a few days and I was getting more excited as the time got closer. The evening before our parents were to come get us we had a party. Of course, the highlight of the party was opening all the presents. I couldn't believe it when Santa Claus handed me that big box wishing me a Merry Christmas. My wish came true. When I opened it, there was a Raggedy Ann doll, just like the one in the stories. I felt so special. After 43 years her face is now stained, her red hair faded, her original clothes quite worn, but, she still has her "I love you" heart painted on her chest.

The Christmas reprieve from the hospital was over too soon. This time I really felt homesick. As the weeks went by, though, I once again settled into the hospital schedule. I was fitted with full-length steel and leather leg braces that locked at the knee. I also wore a corset for back support and walked with two canes. In physical therapy I learned to climb steps by swinging one straight leg slowly up a step and hoisting the other leg up by pulling against the handrail with my strong arm. Since my knees were locked it was easier to go down the steps backwards. I simply held onto the handrail and slid my heels off the steps with the use of my hip muscles one at a time. I was proudest of learning how to get up from the floor without assistance if I fell. Of all the things taught to me in my rehabilitation, that one technique gave me back the most confidence in my body—confidence which had been taken away by the poliovirus.

By the Spring of 1953, the hospital had done its job well. I was ready to go home just before Easter. For the first time since the day I got polio I was afraid. I was leaving the shelter of the hospital life and going back to the real world. The day my parents took me home was quite an occasion. As daddy was helping me get into the car he warned me that people might stare at me. He said I should not let it bother me. I guess he was trying to protect me but it was the beginning of a new self-consciousness that would haunt me for years to come.

My parents and grandparents did everything they could to help me adjust to my new physical limits and still live a full life. They valued education and self-sufficiency. They were hard workers and planned ahead for my brother and me to be independent of them. They taught me to use my head since my body was weak. My parents persuaded the inaccessible Catholic grade school to accept me back so I would not have to go to a special school for "crippled" children. Fourth and fifth grades were on the first floor, but I remember having to climb the two flights of steps every day for sixth grade. The school arranged for a muscular eighth grade boy to carry me down the stairs during fire drills. I was embarrassed, more so out of my budding sexual feelings, but secretly liked the special attention. He would be 55 years old now and I wonder how he remembers the short "crippled" girl he was ordered by the nuns to rescue in case of fire.

My body continued to get stronger with the help of a physical therapist who came to the house once a week. About a year after I went home, I "graduated" from long leg braces to just one knee brace on my right leg. I used one cane and stopped wearing my corset. My left leg could support me without a brace because it locked in place by severe "back-kneeing." At that time, the focus was on how much I could push my own muscles to support me and not on how much I should protect those muscles. (Though, one entry in my diary said that my physical therapist told me I should rest more.) I felt vulnerable and the knee brace cut into my shin, but I persisted in the expected goal of walking without artificial support.

One Sunday afternoon when I was eleven my parents were gone and my grandparents were taking care of my brother and me. They took us to a park. I was able to play on the swing and do a little climbing on the "monkey bars" with help. I wanted to ride on the "merry-go-round," so Grandpa lifted me on. Before I could grab the bar a man came along and put his child on, then gave it a hard spin. I went flying off and landed on the knee without the brace. They carried me home in a lot of pain. I remember lying on the couch at my grandparents' house. I was watching the "Ed Sullivan Show" and trying to keep my mind off how much it hurt until my parents came and decided what to do. Grandpa was hoping it was just sprained, but no such luck. I ended up having to lie in bed for several months in traction. This time my mother was my nurse. Our house was two stories, so it was a lot of exercise for *her* while *my* muscles atrophied. After I was able to start bending my leg again and relearning to walk for the third time, I went back to two long leg braces, which I have worn ever since.

I guess this was when I gave up the goal of walking without braces in favor of feeling safer. I was living a full life of school, Girl Scout activities, and friendships. There were other things I was more interested in doing than concentrating on walking without braces. Besides, I could rely on my Grandma to keep praying for a miracle. Every day I took a sip from the bottle of holy water she got for me from

Lourdes, the Catholic shrine in France where cures from all sorts of diseases happened. I wanted to believe that I could be restored to the way I was, but I started counting on it less and less. Instead, I started the long journey of accepting my body the way it was.

Part II: Maturing With Polio, June/96 to October/97

I turned forty in 1983. I found myself getting more upper respiratory infections, and being tired all the time. Seems like I would just get over a cough then I would get it again a couple months later, even in the summer. I had always counted on my arms as the strongest part of my body; now they were beginning to hurt more and more. I couldn't walk as far as I used to without getting out of breath; the curvature of my spine was getting worse; and I was dragging my right leg more than usual. I even needed to wear glasses to read now! By 1985 I had to make a decision to drop out of many of the advocacy activities I was involved in.

Coincidentally, there appeared in the newspaper an article about a woman who was having physical problems similar to mine after having polio some thirty years before. She was starting a support group in Dallas. With some fear I went to one of the first meetings and discovered that there were many people around my age who were experiencing pain, fatigue, severe loss of muscle functioning and breathing difficulties related to having had polio. Many of them who seemed to have fully recovered from polio were having a return of their original symptoms. We did not know if the original poliovirus flared back up in our bodies or if our new weakness was caused by overuse. We were all afraid of our childhood nightmare returning. I felt overcome by a strong sense of connection with everyone at the meeting. For the first time since childhood, I was with people who were just like me. It was like finding brothers and sisters I did not know I had.

The support group pointed me to the dwindling medical resources in Dallas who knew about polio. I was first evaluated by a local physical therapist who had treated children with polio back in the 1950s. She referred me to an orthotic specialist who encouraged me to trade in my old steel braces for molded lightweight ones. It took a while for me to get used to the way they felt, more like my own legs than heavy cages of support. It was like giving up a favorite broken-down pair of old shoes. But for the first time I had a bigger choice in *what* kinds of shoes I could wear.

A three-wheeled electric scooter did the most for my shrinking energy level for going longer distances. I no longer felt like a "tag-along," having to catch up to people or hold them back. I also consulted a nutritionist who helped me with diet and vitamin supplements to correct my body's inability to properly assimilate protein and to increase my energy. I found some relief from respiratory difficulties by participating in an allergy research study along with some of the polio support group members.

Within five years my health stabilized again. Then I had to deal with another time of crisis that sent me into a tailspin of depression and fatigue. First, my beloved grandparents died within a few months of each other. Then Phil and I decided to get married. He lost his job, soon found another position, and then we bought a house and moved our two households and my office. Almost a year later my mother died.

I was over the top on the Life Changes Stress Scale. I was in mourning. I knew I would eventually stop grieving and come out of "burnout" if I respected my process, but I was afraid the breathing problems and enormous fatigue I was experiencing would debilitate me even further. The next step was to make changes in my daily schedule. There was no way I could keep up the demands of my private practice. So I closed my practice to new clients and saw only four clients until they could stop therapy. This last step was hard because it meant my husband was bearing most of the financial burden. He was willing, as he always is when it comes to my health, to make an extra sacrifice. Over the years of our marriage so far, he has kept the vow that he surprised me with during our wedding ceremony: being my *helper.*

I dropped out of most of my volunteer activities, started going to a therapist for massages, and tried to take more naps. When I would begin to feel a little more energy, I found myself right back overdoing it again. Even though I was more at peace with myself emotionally, overcompensating for not feeling good enough was a hard habit to break. I had to keep reminding myself that *preserving* was more important than *producing* and *being* was more important than *doing*.

I am now in my early 50s and, as I move into this new era of my life, I feel the legacy of my parents and grandparents growing within me. They knew when to be serious and do one's duty, and they knew when to play. They kept going despite their physical pain. They were curious and loved learning. They believed in service and keeping promises. They loved fully and without reservation. They knew how to call forth the best from those they cared about.

I feel a deepening spiritual conviction that living well in my physical body depends more on my *attitude* than on anything I actually do to "fix" my body's imbalances. I am practicing a more Zen approach to my physical wellbeing. I meditate to get some detachment from my everyday pain and stress. I try to view pain as just another aspect of living that I shouldn't try to get away from, since it is futile to even try. I am also practical and take analgesics when meditation isn't enough. I study about nutrition and herbs and ways of moving. I try to arrange my life to economize my energy output. I'm always open to new ideas or handy hints that I get from other polio survivors. I still complain and get angry, especially when I am tired, but I feel a foundation in me of confidence that it won't matter how crippled or ill my body might get, I'll just be a Wise Old Crone then. I look for those models of age and competence to emulate, like Mother Teresa, Katharine Hepburn, Golda Meir, Eleanor Roosevelt, etc. I think about Old Indian Shamen, Yoda in Star Wars, and Japanese artists who are revered as national treasures. I want to be like them.

I have come a long way from the frightened, shy teenager who did not like her body. Even though I still feel awkward in movement when I walk, it surprises me that I can dance with some sense of grace. Last year when I was having lunch with a pastoral counselor friend of mine he was telling me how he was thinking about some of our mutual friends. He imagined what heaven would be like for each of them. When it came to me he said, "Heaven for Joyce would be being able to jitterbug." I laughed thinking it was sweet of him to think about me having a good time like that, but on my way home I found myself starting to work out a jitterbug routine that I felt I could do if I slowed the music down. I thought about the song "In the Mood" and with excitement in my voice I called him up to propose a time we could try it out together. He liked the idea and we performed it in front of our group of friends as a Christmas present to them. I just knew I was going to fall down and break something. I almost backed out of doing it, but he persisted in encouraging me and we had a great time. No one expected it to be perfect. Just doing it at all was a delightfully unexpected surprise. The more I kept my mind on the music, rather than on how my body looked to someone else, the easier it was for me to feel the exhilaration of energy when I danced.

I notice now that my hip could be hurting all day, but when I take the time to put music on and *move with the music*, it doesn't hurt at all. The same is true for sexual activity, laughing, or doing a project that captivates my mind so much that I lose track of time. I guess there is a secret lesson that I learn over and over about the experience of *flow*. I am no different than anyone else who has to learn how to live well on this earth. Having a polio-altered body accentuated this lesson. I am reminded on a minute-by-minute basis that *I am my body* and I am *more* than my body. I can either try to change my body, get away from it by denying what my body needs and concentrate only on intellectual or spiritual pursuits, or I can accept the fullness of my physical reality.

Does post-polio syndrome have any influence on my sexuality? Yes, some. Having had to deal with my new debilitation from polio in my later years, I feel a greater appreciation for my physical body. I like my body. I feel sexy in this body. I feel like I have always wished I could feel as a woman, having been through menopause and feel like I no longer have to *prove* myself as a woman. I graduated through enough sexual experiences with men to know in my very bones that I am *good enough* as a woman whose misshapen body does not match the standard of beauty in our culture. My sexuality is comfortably integrated into the rest of my identity for the time being.

I recognize how precarious the balance of energy is in my life right now and how acutely aware I am of protecting my reserves, so it is easier to make sexual activity a lower priority in the list of things I want to spend my energy on. It's just like how Phil and I are planning for his retirement in the near future. We are weighing the costs versus the benefits of spending, while accumulating more assets and figuring out how we are going to make them last as long as we do. What is an orgasm worth and how do I get the most from it? Post-polio syndrome has made me pay very close attention to how much effort everything takes, and how I can't take for granted anymore that I'll have the energy to complete things I start. Phil and I aren't as flexible or "athletic" as we used to be, so we have had to invent more comfortable positions when we make love. We also take more time with each other and don't try so hard to have a goal. We are thinking less of sex and more of *pleasuring* each other. I am considering even instituting a *pampering weekend* once a month when we would take turns pampering each other, making sure no chores or interruptions dilute this special time together.

Ten years have passed since I started this second go-around with my old enemy, polio. What have I learned? What truths will carry me through the rest of the years I have left? I learned that living well with the deteriorating effects of polio depends more on how I *think* and *feel* than on what I do physically. I can no longer count on my physical health remaining stable for a long period of time. It also takes more to maintain what strength I do have.

I learned not to deny my fragility. When I experience my fragility I experience the paradox of its strength. When I stop comparing what I can do now with what I used to be able to do, I am more nourished by the fullness of *one* thing well done that day. I have learned to think in different terms. When I think of rest as a state of mind, rather than an absence of activity, I have more serenity, composure and calm. Being involved in the disability rights movement gave me a way to think about disability as a subculture and not just a disease. I can feel proud of what I have achieved despite my disability, but my new perspective of my disability shared in a larger context can only make me more whole. Polio is and will be my best teacher.

Joyce Ann Tepley is a licensed clinical social worker who lives in Dallas, TX.

We Have Choices*

Doris Staats

All people have to deal with limitations or handicaps—physical, psychological or emotional. What we must realize is that we have choices of how we will deal with our limitations and what our attitude will be. It's up to us to choose whether we will work towards fulfillment or stagnate in self-pity, bitterness or feelings of hopelessness.

*Previously Published in *Options*.

Four years ago when I began to notice the effects of what has now been diagnosed as post-polio syndrome, I was devastated and felt out of control. Like many of us, I had fought back over 35 years ago and had been riding high on my achievements and productivity. The muscle weakness, pain and fatigue gradually became overwhelming and I was frightened, angry and frustrated.

Soon my emotions were governing my actions and I found myself dwelling on the "illness" and not on wellness. The story could have ended there, if it were not for the loving concern and support of two very special friends. They spent months telephoning, writing, talking and looking for the choices of action that might help me to establish a new direction—a new balance in my life—a way for me to feel the best that I could. They presented the choices, but to try them was left up to me. It was difficult to take the first step. And the second, and then the third. I often became discouraged when a choice dead-ended and I found that it didn't work for me.

I have gradually learned that no one person has all the answers, and to place all my energies and hopes in one choice can lead to pain, frustration and discouragement. I have learned that instead, I can take control of my life by combining some choices, giving them enough time to work or not work, and to keep exploring options.

I've learned that rest can be gained in many different ways and the key is to learn what works best for you. Maybe it can come from shortening your work day, from changing your work environment, from taking naps or from using a wheelchair or scooter for long distances. Regular exercise in a nonstressful manner can do wonders for your energy level and your emotional wellbeing. Swimming and gently stretching on a daily basis have worked for me. What's important is to choose a routine that works best for you.

Controlling the pain brought a greater challenge. I had become addicted to prescribed painkillers and a victim of side effects due to prolonged use. Some of my new choices have been myotherapy trigger-point pressure, whirlpools, chiropractic adjustments, acupuncture and relaxation techniques. Relief doesn't occur overnight. Many of my new choices are now a regular part of my daily, weekly or monthly routine and need to be, in order to achieve their maximum benefit.

Accepting the fact that I needed to use new orthotic devices was both difficult and, at times, devastating. I fought against them until

I realized that they were just another one of my choices. I had the choice of falling or walking, of further damaging my body or taking care of it, and of sitting home or doing the things I enjoy. Once I made the decision, I found an orthotist close to home and worked with him. I didn't hesitate to keep going back for adjustments and told him what was not working for me. We became a working team.

Good nutrition is a choice we don't often talk about. I sought out two nutritionists and with their help I have found a diet, along with vitamin and mineral supplements, that not only controls my weight but has me feeling the best I have felt in years.

The final choices have to do with my emotions, my self-respect and my sense of self-worth. We all have many feelings that need to be dealt with and the choices of how we go about this are numerous. I have tried several, such as professional counseling, support groups, and talking to family members and friends with whom I feel comfortable in sharing my thoughts, feelings, frustrations and, at times, anger. It has been a real discovery to learn that I have choices. Maybe what's important is not always succeeding in them, but in trying them. For in trying them I can still control my life and that gives me hope.

Doris Staats is a retired teacher and former member of the Board of Directors of the Polio Society in Washington, DC and lives in Brandywine, MD.

From Manual to Electric: A Transition*

Hugh Gregory Gallagher

My old manual wheelchair is like the philosophy problem set by Grandpa's ax: "This is Grandpa's ax. Of course the handle has been replaced several times and this is the fourth new blade, but it is still Grandpa's old ax, isn't it?" My manual chair, an E&J Junior, is over 25 years old. Everything on it has been replaced two or three times—even the frame itself. The parts have been recycled but it is my same old chair, battered, hopelessly out of date, but *me*.

My old chair has taken me around the world. It once fell out of the trunk of a car going 70 miles an hour—and survived. In Africa it was

*Published in *New Mobility*, March, 1992.

stepped on by a hippopotamus. Jack Kennedy tripped over it in the U.S. Senate. In Alaska, my chair and I were lashed to a pallet and swung ten stories up and over the North Pacific onto an oil platform. I manipulate my old chair with a skill and precision borne of years of practice. My chair has been an integral part of my life, good days and bad, sickness and health, for more than a quarter century.

I am a polio: my trunk and legs are paralyzed, my shoulders are weak, and my biceps and triceps are not so hot. Advancing age and post-polio syndrome are taking their toll. In recent years, I have lost muscle power and endurance. I must now carefully plan my outings, gauging how far my increasingly limited muscle power can take me. More and more, I have become dependent upon the push-power of my friends to get me out and about in the world. Incrementally yet absolutely, I have become less independent, more invalid.

Clearly, time to think of an electric wheelchair.

I resisted the thought. Electric wheelchairs are for *crippled* people, not for folks like me. In my mind's eye, I am one of those lean, mean athletic wheelies who compete in the marathon and get their pictures on the back of Wheaties boxes. And besides, electric wheelchairs are *so big*, like Sherman tanks, nothing at all like my little lightweight chair, which goes so fast and turns on a dime. And besides, I want to be independent; I can't have my mobility threatened by battery failure. I am not the Energizer Bunny; I am flesh and blood.

Most reluctantly, I began the search for a suitable electric powered chair. This took close to a year. There was something wrong with every model, every brand: too big, too high, too wide, too heavy, too expensive—all of them ugly to my eyes. Finally, thanks to the extraordinary helpfulness of the Invacare Company, I decided on an Invacare 9000, customized to the exact dimensions of my old E&J Junior.

I chose the 9000 because it has certain real advantages. As it is the same size as my old chair, it does not impinge upon my independent lifestyle. I am able to make the same transfers and function in the same way from the new chair as from my old one. Also the 9000 is almost portable: the power unit pulls out and the chair folds. A reasonably strong and determined man can take it apart and put it in the trunk of a car in under three minutes.

It took time to get used to the electric controls. At first, I was a terrible, klutzy driver. I lurched around the house like a drunk in a dodgem car at the carnival. I took the bathroom door off its hinges, not just once but twice. I made holes in the walls. I upset a table and ran into a tree.

I had an attitude problem. Using the 9000, I had—still have—a sense of failure, a sense that I have given up, given in, after all these years of struggle, to my polio paralysis. I had a terrible feeling that, unless I continued to push my muscles each day to their very limits, they would soon waste away, leaving me as not much more than a talking vegetable.

For the longest time, I kept the 9000 in the corner, using it only a few minutes a day. To my mind it was as seductive, dangerous, and habit-forming as drugs are for Nancy Reagan. The 9000 sang a powerful siren song: with it I could do wonderful things, things I have never been able to do in my manual chair. But I just said NO.

Here are some of the wonderful things I did with my 9000:

- I went to the National Gallery in my new electric. For the first time since polio, I was able to look at the pictures at my own speed without worrying about my own effort or fatigue or being dependent upon the sensitivity of the person pushing.
- On my own, I went Christmas shopping at the Mall, stopped for a drink and dinner, and then home again via a lift-equipped taxi van.
- I went for hikes in my electric along the towpath of the C&O Canal National Park. This is a wonderful park that stretches more than 50 miles alongside the Potomac River. From the tow path I have seen turtles sunning, wild deer, a bald eagle and a russet-sided twohee.
- On summer evenings, often with my neighbor, I went for an electric stroll around our community, meeting and chatting with my neighbors for the first time.

I enjoyed all this greatly. It was a liberation for me to go out into the world independent of the strength of my arm muscles. I had not realized just how much in recent years my world had shrunk as my biceps had weakened.

Even though I have used a chair for 40 years, I am still self-conscious when I am out in public. I am still very aware how people react to me in my chair. It is my sense that strangers react slightly differently to me in my electric than they do to me in my manual. I think the manual is perceived as personal equipment—like crutches, or perhaps a blindman's cane. The electric, on the other hand, is seen as a thing—a vehicle something like a golf cart. When you talk to someone in an automobile, he is *inside*, while you are outside. In a way, that is how people talk to me while I am in my electric chair: I am in my vehicle and they are outside it. My manual chair is not such an obstacle; it does not get in the way of conversation as my electric chair does. On the other hand, in motion, the electric chair moves from A to B so effectively, so efficiently that it imparts to its occupant a dignity that is somehow missing in a hand-propelled chair. It is a *very sensible* way to go about your business.

I have had my Invacare 9000 for six months. It has changed my life. I use it full time around the house and I keep my manual folded in the back seat of my car. I no longer struggle with getting my manual in and out of the car. When I am going somewhere, I transfer from the electric to my car and leave the electric standing in the driveway. Using the electric I find I no longer have that deep, almost permanent muscle fatigue I used to drag around with me—or at least not so much. My arm muscles are more rested, and as a result I am able to do transfers better than I have in years. I also do more transfers. My arm muscles have gained strength yet may have lost something in endurance—but it is hard to say for sure.

In sum, I am not a failure, I have not given up, I am just sensible. I am no vegetable. I won't say I lived happily ever after but I will say I have, at last, made the transition from manual to electric. It is a transition I should have made years ago.

Hugh Gregory Gallagher is a writer and historian who lives outside Washington, DC in Cabin John, MD.

Overcoming Overcoming

Carol J. Gill

Two years after contracting polio, I started elementary school. Following doctors' advice, my parents enrolled me in the special education "school for crippled children" that served my region of the city. On the first day of class, I arrived well prepared with a new pencil box, thermos and lunch bag. What I was poorly prepared for, however, was my immersion in a disability community. I dutifully took my assigned seat and, with mounting panic, surveyed my classmates. I saw missing legs, uncontrolled movements, a child writing with her toes and strange equipment everywhere. Immediately, I knew that I had been brought there in error; I certainly did not belong in a room full of cripples.

I had, in fact, been tutored to see myself in quite different terms. Although three of my limbs were paretic, my scoliosis was severe, and I practically lived in heavy leg braces, no one in my family ever uttered a word suggesting I had a disability. Polio was a "sickness" and I was "getting well." My mission in life was to "try harder" and not to give in to my tired muscles. Nothing lay beyond my abilities if I worked hard enough. I learned to see myself not as disabled but as a regular child challenged and inconvenienced by some obstacles to surmount. Sitting in a classroom of authentically disabled children, then, felt like forced abdication. I was angry, sad and scared about its meaning.

Memories of those feelings aided my later work as a clinical psychologist whenever clients with post-polio balked at the idea of joining disability groups. After repeated instances of such resistance, I realized how common it was for polio survivors to view themselves as different from others with disabilities. Seeking the company or support of disabled peers would mean admitting on a deep emotional level that they *had* a disability. That admission could, in turn, unravel all the other tenets of the polio "non-disabled" identity, such as the belief that all things can be accomplished by trying harder, or the taboo against saying "I can't."

Once this realization dawned, it accounted for a lot of behavior I had observed: the shunning of ventilator-using quadriplegic polio survivors by those with less visible disabilities; the lack of interest in disability rights organizing among polio survivors; and the shock and enduring devastation experienced by persons encountering symptoms of post-polio late effects syndrome. As in other minority groups, people who are working overtime to "pass" and assimilate into the dominant culture would naturally feel uncomfortable about both being different, themselves, and publicly affiliating with others who are different, especially if the differences are flagrant. Moreover, they would hesitate to draw attention to their different status by joining a movement for political rights as a distinct group.

This discomfort with minority identity is a direct result of stigma—of learning from the surrounding social environment that being different from the norm is invalidating. We who acquired polio-related disabilities were a broad cross-section of everyday America, most of us children who were "normal" and active one day, confusingly "sick" the next. We were not born "defective," nor were we definitively "maimed" in accidents. We were something else, something less hopeless. Everyday we saw hope in our family's, health professionals', and teachers' eyes that we would never be like the pitiful dependent outcasts who were truly crippled. We learned what we had to do to be valid human beings, namely, overcome our weaknesses and refuse to be disabled.

In that context, modern laws such as the Americans with Disabilities Act (ADA) may provoke some conflict in many polio survivors. The disability rights movement has gathered boldness in its quest for reasonable accommodation. Twenty years ago many activists focused on simple barrier removal so that those whose disabilities did not prevent independent functioning would be free to navigate the environment. They might view it as heretical to ask for help or admit to having inherent limitations. Now, however, activists have stopped apologizing for being different and, instead, criticize society for failing to respond adequately to disability. The laws they promote mandate accommodations from the public, including personal and technological assistance, for disability-related limitations and untraditional modes of functioning.

For those of us carefully taught never to say, "I can't," and to view needing help as pitiful—as "crippled"—the notion of entitlement to accommodation may be little more palatable than trading our crutches for a motorized wheelchair. Yet some of us have made the leap quite dramatically. For example, Johnny Creshendo, a rock singer/songwriter with post-polio who performs in the British Disability Arts Circuit, writes and speaks powerfully about the improvement in his self-esteem when he stopped hiding his disabled leg and decided to identify proudly as a member of the disability activist community. American disability scholars and community leaders with post-polio, such as Irving Zola, Eleanor Smith and

Hugh Gallagher, have critiqued imposed standards of productivity and rugged autonomy that may suit the nondisabled world but may be demeaning and damaging to us.

The disability rights and independent living movements have provided us with the revolutionary notion that disability is a legitimate part of life, and that most of disabled people's problems are not caused by our bodies but by social oppression. The burgeoning disability pride and culture movement goes farther. Its radical message is that differences are to be embraced, not simply tolerated—that the legacy of our struggle is a richness of experience and perspective that can benefit the world. By participating in these movements, persons with disabilities combat stigma by (1) making the world more inclusive, (2) asserting a positive identity, and (3) enjoying the support of the disability community.

The possibility of embracing those disabled parts we have tried so hard to overcome and ultimately learned to hide is an exciting promise of personal integration. To relinquish the strain of trying to be nondisabled and to let go of it deliberately, in celebration, not in disgrace, is a truly liberating idea. Far from giving in or giving up, self-acceptance is an empowering process. It will no doubt require a good deal of unlearning old ways of looking at ourselves and others with disabilities before some of us "successful polios" will relinquish our place on the treadmill of overcoming. But thinking of all the ways we can re-direct that misused energy may inspire us to give it a try. Ironically, accepting ourselves as disabled could heal us in a way more profound than anything envisioned by the March of Dimes.

Carol Gill is an assistant professor and Director of the Chicago Center for Disability Research at the University of Illinois at Chicago.

Tough Love in the 50s, Mainstreaming and Support Groups

Stanley L. Lipshultz

I often have this dream. It is a warm summer day, and I am playing with my six-year-old playmates on a lush, green field of grass. I can feel the blades tickle my feet as I run through them. We are having a grand time. Then, suddenly, I am alone. My friends are gone and I am running up a hill. I can feel a gentle wind caress my face as I reach the crest of the hill. I love the sensation of running. I have my arms outstretched, pretending to be an airplane. I am gliding, effortlessly over the landscape. I can *feel* the muscles in my legs working, moving me along some unmarked path. I get to the top and that is when I wake up. I always wake up. I never get to run down the hill. I cannot get down the hill, at least not without a lot of effort on my part, and not on the same legs that took me to the top. But, I am not upset. Because I can have this dream, because my six-year-old did experience the first part of this dream, I am fortunate. I can't run anymore, and sometimes I can barely walk, but I am still lucky.

My first encounter with polio is still the most vivid one. It started with what everyone thought was the flu, then with my not being able to move my legs, and a trip to Children's Hospital in Washington, D.C. I remember the anguished looks on my parents' faces when they wrapped me in a blanket and put me in our car for the trip to Children's. I sensed (as a child senses) that they were worried, frightened and trying to look brave. Now that I am a parent, I understand their anguish. I had a morbid fear of hospitals and was terrified by the prospect of an operation. I recall being reassured that they weren't going to operate on me. And I remember the doctor telling me that the spinal tap he was going to do wouldn't hurt. It did. It hurt a lot, and I will never forget it. What six-year-old would—or could—forget the physical pain linked with a needle in the back, and afterwards, over the years, what seemed like endless surgeries?

Looking back on my new beginning, I suppose it was not coincidental that I became introverted. I fantasized what it might be like to run, or jump, to play football or baseball with my friends. When I first assumed the mantle of "crippled" in 1950, the fear of the polio epidemics was still uppermost in many minds. I lost many friends and playmates because their parents would not let them spend time with me. Some of those that remained found some delicious satisfaction in poking fun at my braces and the way that I walked with them. I was always the last person chosen for every playground game. The feuds in these games revolved around who would be forced to choose me to be on a team, not which one was going to win or lose. Polio certainly did hamper my athletic abilities.

My first support group was, and to this day remains, my family. My mother and father were always there for me as were my younger brothers, all three of them. Over the years my support group has grown by three because my children like to play the parent with me. My children are concerned about my deteriorating condition and they show it by insisting that I always use my wheelchair. I suppose in a way it is their payback for my having to discipline them when they were growing up. Whoever said, "What goes around comes around," really knew something!

After my stay in the isolation ward, the big polio ward, physical therapy, painted feet on the wooden base of the parallel bars, hot packs, and bracing, I came home. I shared a room with my two brothers who were four years old at the time. I remember being "special" but not much else. I remember that I was not expected to perform the usual stuff that kids do around the house, like mowing the lawn, taking out the trash, walking the dog. I do know I washed more than my fair share of dishes and did other chores that did not require a lot of walking.

No matter, because I did get plenty of support from my family, although what amounted to the tough love of the 50s, *mainstreaming*, was in retrospect, not all that healthy for us polios. We were still expected to *physically* do all that we had done before, just like polio had been a bad dream! Now we know that we should have conserved some of that energy. I still recall the lecture that we polios were just like everyone else (funny I don't recall seeing all that many other people with braces on their legs) and we were expected to take up right where we left off, as if nothing had happened to us. We did just that; but we also went underground, which is why the evolution of the support group over the past 10 years to 15 years has become important to so many post-polios.

What about the early support groups? Well there weren't any that claimed outright to perform that function. The closest thing to a support group was the overnight camp I attended in the Catoctin Mountains in Maryland. Camp Greentop was a camp for *crippled children*. No doubt I was too young to realize that the label "crippled" was not a good thing. I am certain that in these modern, politically correct times many would be chagrined by hearing that term. I was much older when I put two and two together about Camp Greentop, realizing that it was an important turning point in my life. Up until that time, I suppose I had been pretty down about the fact that I was different from my peers and that they reacted to me in a less than positive way. Now I was in a place where my disability put me at the high end of the achievement list, that is, my disability was minor compared to others around me. Being with others who were more severely disabled than I provided me the opportunity to make a very important life choice. I could spend the rest of my days wondering why I had been chosen to be so very "special" and attend one pity party after another. Or, I could be grateful that the disability I had was not as severe as others that I observed. Greentop was a wonderful mixing bowl of disabilities of every type from birth defects to polio to muscular dystrophy and cerebral palsy. I decided to be thankful for the type of disability that had adopted me.

I only have the fondest memories of Greentop. Being with others who were more severely disabled and who took their disabilities in stride helped me make a dramatic life turn, even at my young age. I always thought I was precocious and now, at age 11, I was sure of it. As far as I am concerned Greentop was a prototype of the ideal support group, and I did not even know it at the time.

After my two summers at Camp Greentop, I went completely underground. As I grew older, I found less of a need to compete on a physical level and concentrated on "fitting in" with my peers by using my head. By the time I reached junior high school, polio was no longer feared by the masses, and hence, neither was I! Even though I spent my phys-ed period in the library, I was more readily accepted by my fellow students, since brawn was no longer the only criterion used to determine a person's worth. I have a much more detailed recollection of my junior and senior high school days than elementary school, probably because I was treated as an equal rather than as an outcast.

My early childhood memories after polio are still buried deep in the recesses of my subconscious where they can't hurt me. I followed those mainstreaming rules to the letter. I pretended to be normal and kept up with the best of them. I couldn't play football or basketball, but neither could a lot of kids. Only my best friends in the whole world knew about my disability. I became the consummate *passer*. And I functioned just fine for the longest time. *Passing*, unfortunately, came with a price. Who knew? Being "normal" took an enormous amount of energy, both physical as well as emotional. To this day I often have difficulty accepting the fact that I am disabled and that my disability is getting worse. Some wags might call this *denial.* I call it S.O.P. for polios. First of all, I am disabled, I just don't like to admit it. So, mentally of course, I am attempting to ward off those inner demons—the ones that are constantly reminding me of the source of my problems—and that takes a lot of effort, almost as much effort as it takes to walk. It took me over forty years to accept my disability and learn to coexist with it. It was a high price to pay for passing, and, in retrospect maybe too high a price, as anyone with post-polio syndrome knows.

The next development occurred rather innocently enough. I thought I had noticed a new weakness in my "affected" limb, and I seemed to be tired all the time, especially after walking a few blocks. I went to a hospital in northern Virginia to see if I could get a new orthotic or a brace or something to make walking a little easier. After getting an EMG and a few other tests and attending a "problem conference," I was diagnosed with *aging athletes' syndrome*. I was told to go see a good psychiatrist to assist in dealing with these phantom problems of fatigue, weakness and joint pain. I did nothing. A few years later I read an article in a national news magazine about a doctor at Baylor College of Medicine who had "discovered" and then given a name to a related set of symptoms which appeared 30 years to 35 years after an initial bout of polio. The doctor of course was Lauro Halstead. The article was one of those "good news/ bad news" things. The good news is you are not crazy. The bad news is you have post-polio syndrome. Some message!

Several months after seeing the article on post-polio, my mother called to tell me about the Post-Polio League for Information and Outreach (P-Polio), and gave me a phone number. I spoke to Debby Brewer, who was then the leader of the P-Polios. Debby is a wonderful person and she quickly charmed me into becoming a member of the P-Polio Board of Directors. I did not know what to expect when I attended my first meeting. Of course there was the usual board stuff, but it turned into a support group meeting as well as my coming-out party, all in one. Up until meeting with this group of polio survivors, I don't recall meeting a single person with polio since my Greentop days. The P-Polio group soon became the present day Polio Society.

Coming to that first meeting and talking to others who had polio began a process that made me think about taking off my cloak of invisibility, the one I had draped around me so no one would notice my disability. *Mainstreaming*, by its very nature, forced many polios to go underground and become very good at deception. We are hard to spot. In conversations with most polio survivors, there seem to be a few common themes that run through our personalities. We evolved from *mainstreaming* to become independent (stubborn?) and self-motivated individuals. We are, to some degree, introspective and probably more so than the average non-disabled person. The beginning of the post-polio era had done little to change my attitude toward fighting the syndrome. At least until recently.

What, you might ask, does this prelude have to do with the nature and value of support groups other than the family unit? Well, first, the syndrome brought me out of the closet as a disabled adult. I was forced to deal with the problem because it was starting to noticeably hinder my daily activities. Second, I came in frequent contact with others who had polio. It is an exceptional feeling to be able to share the same life experiences: the quarantine, the polio wards, the hot packs and therapy, the braces, the surgeries. It was exciting. How ironic that post-polio was the source of such excitement! But at least I knew I was no longer the Lone Ranger. Third, the support group members helped me deal, in my own unique and highly contorted way, with my new reality. When I was first diagnosed with post-polio syndrome, I of course decided to handle the new problems the same way I had handled the old, by ignoring the symptoms and pretending they did not exist. What worked for me when I had polio initially, I thought, should certainly work now, and I had gained years of experience in "dealing" with my disability, albeit in all the wrong ways. The post-polio learning curve is considerably longer than the one used for the initial bout of polio. The harder I tried to ignore the post-polio problems, the more pronounced they became. The pain that had always lingered right at the threshold of consciousness was now palpable. There was weakness in my affected leg that I had never noticed before. There was weakness in my unaffected leg that should not have been there. I felt so tired I had trouble concentrating at times. All in all, a set of symptoms that were, to say the least, very alarming. In speaking to others in my support groups, I slowly devised a set of strategies for dealing with post-polio. Thinking back, it is now clear that I could not have dealt with post-polio without our local support groups.

The support group experiences have helped me close the distance between my polio experiences as a child and my polio life as an adult. They have provided me the chance to see more clearly than ever just who that terrified kid was and recognize that some of him is still with me. I have also come to the conclusion that it was easier to deal with acute polio as a child than to deal with post-polio as an adult. When I was six, I had no control over my life. My parents chose the path they believed was best based on what the medical profession had to offer at the time. Now I am facing the same (but also different) disability as an adult and I have more if not total control over what happens. The struggle continues, but it is remarkably easier to handle when you have company.

Stanley L. Lipshultz is a partner in the law firm of Lipshultz and Hone in Silver Spring, MD.

Job Transitions

Sunny Roller with Liina Paasuke

I'm in the process of changing jobs. Again. The thought of a new position in the organization has had me gripped this weekend. I feel like I just swallowed a lead pipe. This is real. I have to move from my comfortable office, really from my current emotional, intellectual and physical comfort zone into the outer space of new interpersonal relationships, new work expectations, and a new physical setting. What lies ahead? Can I handle it? The late effects of polio make all of this more complicated and slightly more confusing.

When we who had polio were growing up, our physicians didn't know enough about polio's late effects to warn us about our career choices. We chose our professions and vocations based on our interests and levels of disability at the time. Many of us never imagined that we'd need to adapt to the changing labor market trends *and* to the alarming late effects of polio as we approached the pinnacles of our chosen careers. We weren't prepared with "an alternate plan B." So, in our mid-life, we are faced with making a wide range of vocational adjustments. We are making job modifications, changing positions, becoming self-employed, or making the decision to enter into an era of retirement and volunteerism much earlier than anticipated. It takes courage to face these changes. And as I focus on new limitations and my vocational options, I muse that maybe all those people who have stopped us on the street and said, "My, aren't you courageous," were right!

So, with lump in throat, we proceed. Something at work has changed. We've changed. It's tough to admit, but a new secondary disability may be playing havoc with our old way of succeeding. The job just doesn't seem to be do-able anymore. It's too strenuous, too stressful, it's just not working out. It is time for a change—some type of job transition. Before we type up a formal resignation in desperation, perhaps we should consider the possibility of a job modification or in the language of the Americans With Disabilities Act (ADA), a "reasonable accommodation." Would it be possible to change a work habit? To purchase a new piece of equipment to help do the job more easily or to create a more flexible work schedule? Many of us need the help of a trained professional, perhaps an occupational therapist or a vocational rehabilitation counselor, to do the creative brainstorming necessary and to help us evaluate our situations objectively. It's important to know our civil rights as they are described in the ADA and individual state civil rights statutes. Many centers for independent living have legal specialists on staff who can provide knowledgeable advice.

Once the alternative strategy for how to modify our job site is identified, the next step is to create a proposal for reasonable accommodation for our employer. At work, it's important to focus on the solution, not on the problem. Carl Menninger who stated that, "Attitude is more important than fact," would likely have advised that it's important to maintain a positive attitude as we compose the proposal. We must believe and feel that we have much to contribute, that a job modification will help us be just as worthy at work as we always were, and that there is no shame in unavoidable physical change. We must remain proud of our ability to adapt, set goals and achieve them by using our ever-present creative flexibility. That's how we have been getting through life with a disability. This is just a new variation on a time-tested theme! Once we have considered and proposed these modifications of our work patterns, the rest is in the hands of our employer. Their decisions will dictate next steps.

But maybe a job accommodation is not appropriate. Maybe it is time to switch jobs completely. People across our country are discovering that no job is guaranteed these days for anyone. Disabled and non-disabled workers alike are experiencing the effects of organizational restructuring, downsizing, and subcontracting. The work is changing rapidly and the worried workforce must follow suit. So, even though our post-polio need for a new line of work may be caused by new endurance issues and muscular weakness, we aren't alone. Additionally, it's good to know that there are many invaluable sources of job seeking/career changing assistance for us. There are private career counselors, counselors at governmental employment security commissions and state rehabilitation agencies, as well as college placement center counselors. There are also rehabilitation counselors and even psychologists to help us deal with any temporary gloom about needing to change. Depression is an important enemy to ward off because it can cause us to underestimate our abilities. Losses need to be put into perspective and our expectations need to become as realistic as possible so we can advance to the next phase in our careers. Many people have joined local job clubs which serve as support groups for individuals as they search for new work. Together people can explore job opportunities with the help of their local resource persons, supported by nearby library computers and the information highway.

As we visualize going to a new job in a new place, it's important to realize that the American workplace is gradually becoming more employee-friendly. Diversity programs, which often include a focus on employees with disabilities, are popping up in many cutting-edge companies. Places of employment are also responding more and more to the needs of women, single parents, under-served racial groups and older workers with flexible scheduling, changing duties, new ways of getting the same job done, and flexible benefits packages. But we still need to speak up and state our needs regarding accommodations. It is imperative to know and exercise our civil rights when it comes to issues such as job design, training, and ongoing vocational support from the very genesis of a new job. The Job Accommodation Network headquartered in Morgantown, West Virginia, is known to be a reputable resource for this type of information (phone: 1-800-JAN-7234).

Changing jobs requires that we know the labor market trends and our own skill levels so we can merge the two successfully. What current labor market leanings can we take advantage of? Which of our skills are transferable or serve as a foundation for a different professional position? I recently read that at businesses like Ford Motor Company workers who were hired for their brawn 20 years ago are now having to use more brain power than muscle power to succeed at work. This is not an unwelcome message to adept polio survivors who have been required to emphasize the power of the intellect over the power of the physique—often on a daily basis.

Some individuals dream of becoming self-employed, which is another option. Working at home is a developing trend, but there are cautions. Such an arrangement can be capital- and labor-intensive. One must also be very self-disciplined, willing to be relatively isolated at home, and willing to take risks. Some counselors advise that such work should strictly be supplemental to a more secure primary income, at least at first. They also suggest that if one really wants or needs to work at home, this arrangement could become a reasonable accommodation for a current, more traditional job that is performed at the company's worksite.

As we consider additional transition options, perhaps retirement or early retirement and volunteerism come to mind. Do you want to retire early? If so, why? This is a critical question to ask. Have all the other options been weighed? Or does it sound like a fast way to escape the problem that polio's late effects has presented? It's important to think through the entire job transition process before making this important decision. Some people take a hiatus to regroup and reflect on what to do next. Some time off work. An extended sabbatical or vacation. Perhaps a medical leave of absence. Would that be affordable and useful? A time to take stock before taking steps.

Another tactic to facilitate a time out is to apply for social security disability income (SSDI) benefits and for social security supplemental income (SSI). Frequently these benefits are coordinated with employee long-term disability plans. This can be a psychologically difficult decision, but it does not have to be a permanent one. One can use this time to explore career choices or develop new skills and then to re-enter the workforce utilizing the work incentive provisions of these programs. If working full time is not an option, working part time to supplement your benefits might be. Obtaining accurate benefit information is critical to assessing these options.

Volunteerism is also a viable option when we consider staying as productive as possible for as long as possible through our mid- and late-life years. A major consideration is choosing organizations that will give us what we need and want in proportion to what we give to the organizations. Pacing ourselves is important for polio survivors who are volunteer contributors and energy conservation remains a priority throughout our retirement years. In any case, it is critical that we engage in activities which are meaningful for us—whether it is volunteer activity or discovering a new hobby. The adventure of self-discovery is ongoing. There are options. We need to take control.

I am indeed in the process of changing jobs. Again. I suspect this job transition won't be my last one. It does take courage to face these changes. But it also requires information-gathering, contemplation, decisiveness, optimism, wisdom, and action.

Sunny Roller is a Research Project Manager and Research Fellow at the University of Michigan Medical Center. She lives in Ann Arbor, MI. Liina Paasuke is a Certified Rehabilitation Counselor with the Michigan Jobs Commission Rehabilitation Services and lives in Ann Arbor, MI. She was the vocational rehabilitation counselor who helped Sonny Roller make the transition to her new job.

How I Learned to Make Peace With My Disability

Nancy Baldwin Carter

The changes began in my thirties. At first it was merely a matter of fatigue. I'd leave early whenever possible, so that I didn't have to travel on the same day I gave a workshop or seminar. Even then, it became harder and harder to sustain the energy level necessary to get people as involved as I wanted to do. I could not get away from the pain that tore through my body, particularly in my head, back, and shoulders. I spent more and more time in bed, eliminating activities that stole strength from my work. Finally, I couldn't do it anymore. The long hours, vigorous "performances" required for the workshops and seminars, tedious stretches on the road, plus all of the regular demands of an adult education program administrator—

every bit of this took more than I had to offer. I had to give up the profession that I loved.

Somehow I knew this had to do with polio. I contracted total-body spinal and bulbar polio when I was eleven. In time, I experienced a good recovery in my legs and left arm, but many muscles in my neck did not return, making it difficult to support my head. As I grew older, I found myself resorting to a trick I had devised to allow my good left arm to supply the muscle power my neck seemed to be losing: I held the back of my neck with my left hand, which lifted my chin and created "breathing space" in my throat. Aside from this, though, I thought I functioned pretty much like everyone else. These new problems baffled me.

Switching to a sedentary job seemed sensible. Luckily, I was able to land a position keeping books in my father's law firm. Less time on my feet. Less required of me all around. Working outside the profession that I had found so rewarding was dull, but I considered this the price I had to pay to accommodate my irritatingly uncooperative physical condition. I thought I could tap dance for time, do a little diversionary waltz clog to earn a bit of cash while buying some peace for my body. It worked, too. Everything settled down.

Unfortunately, it didn't last. Almost imperceptibly, fatigue returned. Exhaustion blended into weakness that somehow produced pain. I couldn't walk more than a block or two. Driving caused a good deal of agony in my back and shoulders and head. I couldn't stand up for more than a few minutes. At home, my hands would no longer let me peel vegetables, for instance, and the distress in my back prevented vacuuming or making a bed.

I sought professional help. Doctor after doctor sent me down a useless path. I saw an unbelievable seven physicians, each one diagnosing his own specialty—the rheumatologist said I had arthritis, while the orthopedist was sure that poor posture was the culprit. Finally, Dr. Ann Bailey in Warm Springs, Georgia, identified post-polio syndrome (PPS). I took her diagnosis and recommendations to my local physician, who scoffed at her suggestions to change my lifestyle. He called the entire PPS theory ridiculous. He said that he, himself, had contracted polio as a young man and that he was fine. He wrote something on a prescription pad and handed it to me saying, "This is someone who will help you." It was the name of a psychiatrist. That did it: I knew then that only I could be responsible for my wellbeing. I had to learn to be assertive and develop a partnership with doctors that worked toward my own best interests. I began the search for an M.D. who was willing to listen and to include me in planning for my care.

All the while, my body continued its slow but steady downward spiral. I stopped working. Though I wasn't able to engage in any significant gainful activity, I didn't see myself as disabled. I knew people who were disabled. They had problems I didn't have. Denial. With everything that was in me, I did not want to be disabled. The word itself was repugnant to me. It meant defeat, hopelessness, the end. I refused to be disabled. I may have been using a wheelchair, unable to complete household tasks, struggling with breathing and swallowing, but by God, *I was not disabled.*

Then I realized if I were going to apply for Social Security Disability Insurance (SSDI), it would have to be soon. I had been encouraging others in our polio association to seek Social Security disability status, and I knew the time parameters. I had to have worked twenty out of the past forty quarters (five of the past ten years), and my time was running out; I had not held a job in over four years. It was a struggle. I had to take a good look at myself and face my fears. To do this, I had to surrender, change my attitude. In the end, maybe still a little reluctantly, I had to concede I was disabled. Once done, however, I had no time for mourning. Getting into the Social Security disability program required all of my attention.

I began by talking with others who had been through the process. Almost everyone said they were turned down initially and then appealed again and again, sometimes spending up to two years before they advanced to the administrative law judge, who granted their claims. It was clear that tenacity was important here. If applicants quit when their claims were first rejected, the process stopped there. Sticking with it often brought them to someone with more understanding and authority to make a favorable decision. As I questioned these people, however, I noticed they all left most of the work up to their doctors. They trusted the doctors to supply the correct information. Considering what I had already learned about looking out for my own welfare, I suspected that this was not a wise approach. This was confirmed when I spoke with a man who had worked with disability claims for the Social Security Administration (SSA). He said that of qualified applicants who are denied SSDI, *the main reason for the refusal is that those involved do not present sufficient details to substantiate a claim for disability.*

Reading everything I could find about getting Social Security disability benefits, I discovered what I needed to do. Time was a big factor. My end of the operation had to be completed soon, and the doctor had only a narrow period in which to finish his part. I began by listing all of my impairments and limitations. I filled out my application as thoroughly as possible, leaving nothing out, no matter how small. While one condition alone may not be enough to qualify a person for disability, the sum may. I copied my application and took it to my doctor along with pages from the Social Security Administration's *Program Operations Manual System* so that he could see how SSA references post polio.

I asked him to write a strong, two-or-three page, fact-filled letter for me to show how I am disabled, to itemize my fatigue and weakness and pain, and to indicate how it interferes with my daily life. I hoped he would talk about such details as my inability to sit and type for more than five minutes without great pain in my neck and shoulders, or that I could not lift more than five pounds, or other similar specifics for activities such as climbing, kneeling, handling objects, and reaching. Phrases such as "persistent fatigue" or "on a daily (hourly?) basis" would show that my problems were beyond the norm for someone my age. Mentioning my "wasting syndrome" and that I was weaker each time my doctor saw me would provide good clues about my PPS.

I requested that he discuss any specific tests, studies, X-rays that verified my disability (e.g., What did my EMG reveal? What were the results of my muscle tests? What were the number of degrees of range of motion of involved joints compared to normal? What were the specifics of my pulmonary tests? What did my swallowing tests indicate? What X-rays illustrated details of my case?).

I reminded him that Social Security is not interested in hearing *his opinion* of whether or not I am disabled; they want only *the facts* so that they can decide the question. I asked for a copy of his letter. I promised to call his office to be sure that his secretary didn't miss the deadline for returning this to SSA. I could see that my doctor was not exactly used to this approach, but he was becoming accustomed to me and went along with it. The important thing to me was that I had input in the process; we did this together. The only other significant step involved my being examined by a doctor employed by Social Security. My claim was approved shortly after I submitted it. I believe that such quick success was because I had done my homework and had decided to put my energy into preparing the initial application rather than in appeals.

Now I am officially disabled. It's not such a bad deal. My body is no different for being called disabled—it's going to be the way it is no matter how I characterize it. But my mind has changed. Acceptance allows me to feel good about who I am and to get on with the positive aspects of living. Sometimes I surprise myself.

Nancy Baldwin Carter is the Founder and Former Director of the Nebraska Polio Survivors Association and lives in Omaha, NE.

Managing Post-Polio Additional Reading and Resources

Chapter One: Acute Polio and Post-Polio Syndrome

Additional Reading

Black, Kathryn. *In the Shadow of Polio: A Personal and Social History*. New York: Addison-Wesley, 1996.

Bodian, D. *Poliomyelitis: Pathological Anatomy, in Poliomyelitis: Papers and Discussions Presented at the First International Poliomyelitis Conference*. Philadelphia, PA: Lippincott, 1949; 62.

Dalakas, MC, Bartfeld, H, Kurland, LT, eds. *The Post-Polio Syndrome: Advances in the Pathogenesis and Treatment*. Annals of the New York Academy of Sciences, 1995; 753.

Gallagher, H.G. *FDR's Splendid Deception* (rev. ed.). Arlington: Vandamere Press, 1998.

Gawne, AC, Halstead, LS. Post-Polio Syndrome: Historical Perspective, Epidemiology and Clinical Presentation. *Neuro Rehab*, 1997; 8:73–81.

Gould, Tony. *A Summer Plague: Polio and Its Survivors*. New Haven, CT: Yale University Press, 1995.

Jubelt, B, Drucker, J. Post-Polio Syndrome: An Update. *Semin Neurol*, 1993; 13(3): 283–290.

Mulder, DW, Rosenbaum, RA, Layton, DD. Late Progression of Poliomyelitis or Forme Fruste Amyotrophic Lateral Sclerosis. *Mayo Clin Proc*, 1972; 47, 756–760.

Paul, John R. *A History of Poliomyelitis*. New Haven, CT: Yale University Press, 1971.

Smith, Jane S. *Patenting the Sun: Polio and the Salk Vaccine*. New York: Morrow, 1990.

Strebel, PM, Sutter, RW, Cochi, SL, et al. Epidemiology of Poliomyelitis in the United States One Decade after the Last Reported Case of Indigenous Wild Virus Associated Disease. *Clin Infect Dis*, 1992; 14:568–579.

Trojan, DA, Cashman, NR. Pathophysiology and Diagnosis of Post-Polio Syndrome, *Neuro Rehab*, 1997; 8:83–92.

Weichers, DO. Late Effects of Polio: Historical Perspectives, in *Research and Clinical Aspects of the Late Effects of Poliomyelitis,* Halstead, LS and Weichers, DO, eds. White Plains, NY: March of Dimes Birth Defects Foundation, 1987; 23(4): 1–11.

Chapter Two: New Health Problems in Persons with Polio

Additional Reading

Agre, JC, Rodriquez, AA, Harmon RI. Strengthening Exercise Can Improve Function in Post-Polio Subjects Without Detectable Adverse Affect Upon the Surviving Motor Units or Muscle. Abstract. *Arch Phys Med Rehab*, 1995; 76:1036.

Auroy, Y, Narchi, P, Messiah, A, et al. Serious Complications Related to Regional Anesthesia: Results of a Prospective Study in France. *Anesthesiology*, 1997; 87:479–486.

Bruno, RL, Cohen, JM, Galaski, T, et al. The Neuroanatomy of Post-Polio Fatigue. *Arch Phys Med Rehabil*, 1994; 75:498–504.

Bach, JR, Alba, AS. Pulmonary Dysfunction and Sleep Disordered Breathing as Post-Polio Sequelae: Evaluation and Management. *Ortho*, 1991; 14:1329–1337.

Dalakas, MD, Elder, C, Hallet, M, et al. A Long-Term Follow-Up Study of Patients with Post-Poliomyelitis Neuromuscular Symptoms. *N Engl J Med*, 1986; 314:959–963.

Gawne, AC, Pham, BT, Halstead, LS. Electrodiagnostic Findings in 108 Consecutive Patients Evaluated in a Post-Polio Clinic: The Value of Routine Electrodiagnostic Testing, in *The Post-Polio Syndrome: Advances in the Pathogenesis and Treatment*, Dalakas, MC, Bartfeld, H, Kurland, LT, eds. Annals of the New York Academy of Sciences, 1995; 753, 353–385.

Gawne, AC Halstead, LS. Post-Polio Syndrome: Pathophysiology and Clinical Management. *CRC Rev Rehab*, 1995; 7:147–188.

Grimby G, Hedberg M, Henning GB. Changes in Muscle Morphology, Strength and Enzymes in a 4–5-Year Follow-Up of Subjects with Poliomyelitis Sequelae. *Scand J Rehab Med*, 1994; 26:121–130.

Gyermek, L., Increased Potency of Nondepolarizing Relaxants after Poliomyelitis. *J Clin Pharmacol*, 1990; 30:170–173

Halstead, LS, Grimby, G. eds. *Post-Polio Syndrome*. Philadelphia: Hanley and Belfus, 1995.

Perry J, Fountain JD, Mulroy S. Findings in Post-Poliomyelitis Syndrome. *J Bone Joint Surg*, 1995; 77-A:1148–1153.

Smith, LK, McDermott, K. Pain in Post-Poliomyelitis: Addressing Causes Versus Treating Effects. In: Halstead, LS. Weichers, DO, eds. *Research and Clinical Aspects of the Late Affects of Poliomyelitis.* White Plains, NY: March of Dimes Birth Defects Foundation, 1987; 125–134.

Sonies, BC, Dalakas, MC. Dysphagia in Patients with the Post-Polio Syndrome. *N Engl J Med*, 1991; 324:1162–1167.

Stalberg, E and Grimby, G. Dynamic Electromyography and Muscle Biopsy Changes in a 4-Year Follow-Up Study of Patients with a History of Polio. *Muscle Nerve*, 1995; 18:699–707.

Trojan, DA, Cashman, NB. *Current Trends in Post-Poliomyelitis Syndrome.* New York, NY: Milestone Medical Communications, 1996.

Waring, WP, Maynard, F, Grady, W, et al. Influence of Appropriate Lower Extremity Orthotic Management on Ambulation, Pain, and Fatigue in a Post-Polio Population. *Arch Phy Med Rehab*, 1989; 70:371–375.

Windebank, AJ, Litchy, WJ, Daube, JR, et al. Lack of Progression of Neurologic Deficit in Survivors of Paralytic Polio: A 5-Year Prospective Population-Based Study. *Neurology*, 1996; 72:729–733.

Chapter Four: How to Find Expert Medical Care

Resources

- American Academy of Neurology
  1080 Montreal Avenue
  St. Paul, Minnesota 55116
  http://www.aan.com
  (612) 695-1940
- American Academy of Orthopaedic Surgeons
  6300 North River Road
  Rosemont, Illinois 60018-4262
  http://www.aaos.org
  (847) 823-7186 or (800) 346-AAOS
  FAX (847) 823-8125
- American Academy of Physical Medicine and Rehabilitation
  One IBM Plaza
  Suite 2500
  Chicago, Illinois 60611-3604
  http://www.aapmr.org
  (312) 464-9700
  FAX (312) 464-0227

- Gazette International Networking Institute/International Polio Network
  4207 Lindell Boulevard, #110
  St. Louis, MO 63118-2915
  www.post-polio.org
  (314) 534-0475
  A good place to start for information. Provides written material about post-polio syndrome; publishes an international directory of support groups, health professionals, and clinics serving polio survivors; sponsors international conferences about post-polio issues; and publishes a quarterly newsletter called "Polio Network News," available by subscription.
- The Polio Society
  4200 Wisconsin Avenue, NW
  Suite 106273
  Washington, DC 20016
  http://www.polio.org
  E-mail address jshl@mhg.edu
  (301) 897-8180
  Provides medical and other information to the public and to health care professionals; sponsors national conferences about post-polio issues; publishes a quarterly newsletter; and sponsors support group meetings in the Washington, DC area.

Chapter Five: Energy Conservation

Resources

On the Internet

- Grace Young's Energy Conservation Web Site. A new topic each month relating to energy conservation. www.geocities.com/HotSprings/4713.

Adaptive Equipment:

- Functional Solutions for Independent Living. North Coast Medical, Inc. (800) 821-9319
- Enrichments. Sammons Preston Inc. (800) 323-5547
- Consumer-Direct Ordering. Smith and Nephew Rolyan. (800) 558-8633
- Abledata. A product database for disability-related products. (800) 227-0216
- Guide to Independent Living. Arthritis Foundation. (800) 283-7800

Home Modifications:

- The DoAble, Renewable Home. A guide to help adapt your home as your needs change. Order from AARP Fulfillment, 1909 K St. NW, Dept. GP; Washington, D.C. 20049. Pamphlet D12470.

- Planning for Access: A Guide to Planning and Modifying Your Home. Eastern Paralyzed Veterans Association. (800) 444-0120
- An Accessible Home of Your Own. Accent Special Publications; Cheever Publishing Inc.; P.O. Box 700; Bloomington, IL 61702.
- Ideas for Making Your Home Accessible. Accent Special Publications; address above.

Vacation/Leisure:

- Air Carrier Access Act: Common Questions and Answers About Air Travel for Wheel-Chair Users. Eastern Paralyzed Veterans Association; 75-20 Astoria Blvd., Jackson Heights, NY 11370-1178.
- Access Travel: Airports. 48-page pamphlet which details facilities, services and accessible design features of airport terminals worldwide. Write the Consumer Information Center; Pueblo, CO 81009.
- New Horizons: Information for the Air Traveler with a Disability. Published by U.S. Dept of Transportation. Write Consumer Information Center; Pueblo CO 81009.
- Adapted Car Rentals. Rental cars with hand controls are available at most airports and major cities. To reserve ahead call: AVIS (800) 331-1212; HERTZ (800) 654–3131; NATIONAL (800) 328-4567.
- Wheelers. To rent wheelchair accessible vans, call (800) 456-1371.

Recreation:

- Access to Recreation. Call (800) 634-4351 for free catalog of adapted recreation equipment.
- Products to Assist the Disabled Sportsman. Write J. L. Pachner; PO Box 164; Trabuco Canyon, CA 92678.

Chapter Six: Lifestyle Changes: Taking Charge

Additional Reading

Smith, LK, Mabry, M.: Poliomyelitis and the Post-Polio Syndrome. *Neurological Rehabilitation*, Umphred, D. ed., 3rd Edition, St. Louis: Mosby, 1995.

Post-Polio Syndrome: *A New Challenge for the Survivors of Polio*. 1997. CD requiring CD ROM Drive, Macintosh or Windows 3.0 or higher. International Polio Network, 4207 Lindell Blvd., Suite 110, St Louis, MO. 63108-2915. Phone: 314/534-0475, Fax: 314/534-5070.

Trojan, D., Cashman, N.B.: *Current Trends in Post Poliomyelitis Syndrome*. New York: Milestone Medical Communications 1996. Available from International Polio Network. Phone: (314) 534-0475.

The Late Effects of Poliomyelitis—an Overview. Questions and Answers about the Post-Polio Syndrome. A publication of the International Polio

Network, 4207 Lindell Boulevard, #110, St. Louis, MO 63118-2915; (314) 534-0475.

Chapter Seven: Psychosocial Demensions of Polio and Post-Polio Syndrome

Additional Reading

Fine, Michelle, Asch, Adrienne eds. *Women with disabilities: Essays in psychology, culture, and politics*. Philadelphia: Temple University Press, 1988.

Finger, Anne. *Past due: A story of disability, pregnancy and birth*. Seattle, WA: Seal Press, 1990.

Fries, Kenny. *Body, remember: A memoir*. New York: Dutton, 1997.

Gallagher, Hugh. *FDR's Splendid Deception* rev. ed. Arlington: Vandamere Press, 1998.

Mairs, N. *Waist high in the world: A life among the nondisabled*. Beacon Press, 1997.

Olkin, R.J. *Treating Clients with Physical Disabilities: An Approach Based on Family Systems and the Minority Model of Disability*. New York: Guilford Press (in press).

Rogers, Judi, & Matsumura, M. *Mother to be: A guide to pregnancy and birth for women with disabilities*. New York: Demos Publications, 1991.

Zola, Irving. *Missing pieces: A chronicle of living with a disability*. Philadelphia, PA: Temple University Press, 1982.

Zola, Irving ed. *Ordinary lives: Voices of disability and disease*. Cambridge, MA: Applewood Books, 1982.

Chapter Nine: Journeying Together: Post-Polio Support Groups

Additional Reading

Bernstein, S. ed. *Explorations in Group Work*. Boston: Boston University, 1962.

Chapter Ten: Vocational Strategies

Additional Reading

Bolles, Richard. *The Three Boxes of Life*. Berkeley, CA: Ten Speed Press, 1981.

Bower, Sharon Anthony, Bower, Gordon H. *Asserting Yourself, A Practical Guide for Positive Change.* Addison Wesley Publishing Co., 1976.

Crystal, John C. and Bolles, Richard. *Where Do I Go from Here with My Life?* Berkeley, CA: Ten Speed Press, 1974.

Thomas, Roberts; Lewis, Janet; Jensen, Nancy. *Job Seekers' Guide to Employment.* San Diego: Regain/Job Seekers' Publications, 1994.

Resources

Organizations providing information and assistance with job and school accommodations are:

- Abledata (NARIC)—(800) 346-2742; http://www.abledata.com
  A national database of information on assistive technology and rehabilitation equipment available from domestic and international sources.
- Adaptability—(800) 243-9232
  A national organization providing lists of equipment and supplies for all aspects of physical needs for disabled persons.
- Job Accommodation Network (JAN)—(800) 526-7234
  An international non-profit information and referral service of the President's Committee on Employment of People with Disabilities since 1983.
- National Rehabilitation Information Center (NARIC)—(800) 346-2742.
  Provides quick reference and referral through an information specialist for all issues including funding possibilities, local agencies, etc. Also includes REHABDATA searches with a descriptive listing of all of the documents at NARIC on a particular topic or combination of topics and ABLEDATA searches. NARIC makes photocopies of documents in their collection available.
- Occupational Outlook Handbook. US Department of Labor, Bureau of Labor Statistics, Washington, DC: 1996–97 ed. Revised every few years. To order write: US Government Printing Office, Superintendent of Documents, Mail Stop: SSOP, Washington, DC 20402-9328.
- The Trace Research and Development Center (University of Wisconsin)—(608) 262-6966. A rehabilitation research institute on adaptive computers and information systems. Website—http:TRACE.wisc.edu. Primarily a research institute on technology and disability, the Center offers a packet of information on computer access. The website offers more information about on-going research & design projects, consumer information and participatory discussions.
- Job Seekers' Guide to Employment, Job Seekers' Publications, San Diego, CA (619) 298-7565. A workbook to assist disabled workers and others to gain entry into new jobs and careers.

Chapter Eleven: Navigating the Managed Care Maze

Additional Reading

Korczwyk, S., Wittey, H., *The Complete Idiot's Guide to Managed Health Care*. New York: Alpha, MacMillan, 1998. (800) 428-5331.

Resources

- American Association of Health Plans, Washington, D.C. (202) 778-3200.
- Managed Care Glossary, Albany, NY: CapitalHealth Publishing, Inc., 1997. (518) 465-2953.
- Managed Care Services, AAPA News, American Academy of Physician Assistants, Alexandria, VA, (703) 836–2272.
- National Committee for Quality Assurance, Washington, D.C. (202) 955-3500.
- Research Activities, Agency of Health Care Policy Research, Center for Information Dessemination, 2101 East Jefferson Street, Suite 501, Rockville, MD 20802. (301) 594-1364.

Chapter Twelve: Playing the Social Security Benefits Card

Resources

- *Guidelines for the Late Effects of Polio*, SSA Document 64-039, Local Social Security Administration office or national office at: (800) 772-1213
- *SSDI: Getting It*, SSA Document 05-10153, Local Social Security Administration office or national office at: (800) 772-1213.

Chapter Thirteen: A Guide to the Internet for Polio Survivors

Additional Reading

Reed KL, Cunningham S: *Internet Guide For Rehabilitation Professionals*. Philadelphia: Lippincott, 1997.

Index

S